# REPORT 2008

## A MAN'S GUIDE TO WOMEN

## BUILT FOR SEX

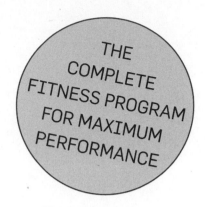

THE COMPLETE FITNESS PROGRAM FOR MAXIMUM PERFORMANCE

# REPORT 2008
## A MAN'S GUIDE TO WOMEN
# BUILT FOR SEX

# Scott Hays

RODALE

First published in paperback in 2005 as *Built for Sex: The Complete Fitness Program for Maximum Performance*

© 2005 by Scott Hays

Printed in the United States of America
Rodale Inc. makes every effort to use acid-free ♾, recycled paper ♻.

Book Design by Susan P. Eugster

Illustrations by Craig L. Kiefer & Kimberly A. Martens
Photographs by Mitch Mandel/Rodale Images

ISBN 13 978–1–59486–874–0 paperback
ISBN 10 1–59486–874–3 paperback

2  4  6  8  10  9  7  5  3  1   paperback

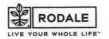

RODALE
LIVE YOUR WHOLE LIFE™

We inspire and enable people to improve their lives and the world around them

For more of our products visit **rodalestore.com** or call 800-848-4735

## SEX AND VALUES AT RODALE

We believe that an active and healthy sex life, based on mutual consent and respect between partners, is an important component of physical and mental well-being. We also respect that sex is a private matter and that each person has a different opinion of what sexual practices or levels of discourse are appropriate. Rodale is committed to offering responsible, practical advice about sexual matters, supported by accredited professionals and legitimate scientific research. Our goal—for sex and all other topics—is to publish information that empowers people's lives.

# CONTENTS

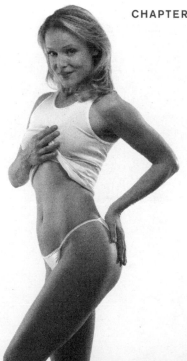

# ACKNOWLEDGMENTS

**THIS BOOK COULD NOT HAVE BEEN WRITTEN WITHOUT THE SUPPORT AND ENCOURAGEMENT OF SEVERAL INDIVIDUALS IN MY LIFE.** I wish to extend my deepest appreciation to all of them, especially my girlfriend of nearly a decade, Marty, who's the only one who can truly appreciate what it's like to live with someone like me.

For his insights into strength conditioning and sex, I'd like to thank personal fitness trainer and consultant Don Alessi of AlessiFit.com. For the eating plan and nutritional analysis, special thanks to Kathleen Hanuschak, RD. For their research and editing skills, I'd like to thank Adrienne Kreger-May and Leah Flickinger at Rodale, and Kevin Jeys, Taran March, and Nan Kappeler. For his research into how many calories it takes to keep a body fit, I'd like to thank Lou Schuler, author of *The Testosterone Advantage Plan*.

# THE BLOODFLOW FACTOR

**IF YOU'VE EVER SPENT ANY TIME AT A GYM, YOU'VE SEEN HIM. PERHAPS (WE HOPE NOT) YOU EVEN ARE HIM.**

We're talking about the guy who goes to the gym, suits up, and then goes around making chin music to everyone else in the place. Sometimes he'll do a couple of stretches or a few half-hearted lifts or maybe take a desultory stroll on the treadmill. But most of the time, he beats his gums. And most important of all, he never—repeat, never—breaks a sweat.

Now do you know who we're talking about? It's not just that he's not serious. It's the way he always gets in your way. Like when you're trying to work through a few sets of weights, and he's using the leg-press machine as a La-Z-Boy.

We're being pretty hard on the poor guy, but only to emphasize that motivation is the key to having great sex. Every one of us, including this dope at the gym, is a collection of habits. Who we are, how we look, and how we perform in bed are in many ways products of that collection. If, for example, your particular collection of habits includes frequent trips to the kitchen between innings on TV, it's a pretty safe bet that you aren't in the best shape of your life. If you always have sex in the same position or come after a certain length of time, chances are you're going to keep doing it unless you put out the energy to change. And that takes work, commitment, and a *desire* to change.

Unless you're willing to devote enormous time and effort to working out, you are probably never going to have abs like the washboards you see on male fashion models. Hard work and dedication will get you fit—fitter than you've ever been in your life. But you won't get that "shredded" look unless nature designed you that way in the first place.

The same is true of penis size, or how often you can make love in a night, or how often you even want to make love. Your lifestyle—how well you eat, how much you exercise, and so on—can certainly prime the pump and make you feel sexy. It can give you the stamina you need for good sex. It can make you sexy to others. But it won't turn you into some kind of Hollywood sex-puppy. That's not realistic. Nor, for that matter, is it necessary.

## A REAL PLAN FOR REAL MEN

When we were researching this book, we talked to a lot of you guys. As you'll see in later chapters, you had a lot of enlightening stuff to say. For starters, you told us you wanted better sex but didn't want to work too hard. The good news is, you don't really have to. Yes, changing your lifestyle and paying attention to the little things takes work, but you're already closer than you think to being attractive to women and having a steamy sex life. How do we know this? When researching the book, we also asked the people who care about how you look and what you do in bed—women. You'll find their voices throughout this book, too. They told us, again and again, that they don't want a man who looks like he lives in a gym. That ripped male physique? It leaves them cold. What they really want is a man who cares enough about himself to stay fit, who can find his way around the kitchen without getting lost, who knows the differences between acrobatic, show-off sex and truly intimate (and hot) encounters.

Six-pack abs and bulging biceps? *"No way!"* a 25-year-old graduate student in New York City told us. *"A guy who's in that kind of shape spends way too much time in front of the mirror. I care about a man's inner beauty, his charm and charisma. That's what makes him sexy."*

The *Built for Sex* plan is based on one simple premise: Every man, whatever his age, diet, or level of fitness, can improve his sex life by making *minimal* changes in his life. Take a moment to let that sink in. You don't need to work out day and night. You don't need to become a vegetarian. You don't have to spend a month's salary on how-to sex books (though the photographs are certainly worth a look). All you have to do is find in yourself the motivation to *tweak* your life rather than turn it upside down.

Here's an example. Doctors who specialize in male sexual problems see a lot of guys who don't get as hard as they'd like. Sure, you can shell out about $10 for a single dose of Viagra or spend a year on a psychologist's couch. But first, try two things and two things only: Improve your diet, and exercise most days of the week. The research is very clear that men who do these two things have better bloodflow, more energy, and enhanced libido. That's one heck of a payoff for two easy changes. Add a couple more tweaks, such as exercises to boost stamina or techniques to intensify orgasms, and the payoff will be even better.

Here are the nuts and bolts of the *Built for Sex* plan. We cover each of these topics in a *lot* more detail later on, but these are the basics.

## STEP 1: HONE YOUR TECHNIQUE

We're all creatures of habit. If you've been with the same partner for a long time, you've probably settled into a comfortable routine: A little kissing, a little foreplay, the same sexual positions. There's certainly nothing wrong with familiarity. Couples usually make love in the same ways because they like the way they feel. On the other hand, sexual ruts can be a real stumbling block if they arise more from routine than from real desire.

A lot of the how-to sex guides seem to assume that every man has joints of rubber and the strength to stand on his head, caress his partner, and have mind-blowing sex all at the same time. In real life, though, few of us have the energy (or the interest) to turn the pursuit of pleasure into bedroom gymnastics. What you can, and should, do is occasionally shake things up in bed. Novelty is a tremendous aphrodisiac.

**TALK OFTEN, IN AND OUT OF BED.** It's hard for men as well as women to say clearly what they want in bed, especially if the things they want seem a little out there. Hey, your partner isn't a mind reader. Sure, a well-timed moan or a little bit of hand pressure speaks volumes about what's working. But you'll never know exactly what your partner wants you to do, or what you want her to do to you, unless you speak up.

Do you want more strength and pressure when she plays with you? Tell her. Do you prefer aggressive oral sex or light touches and teasing? Say so. Do you have fantasies about being totally passive—or, conversely, taking total control? Talk about it. Each man and woman has different desires, different likes and dislikes. Don't leave it all to chance.

**TRY ALL-DAY FOREPLAY.** Sex doesn't begin when you turn out the lights. Couples who report being happiest with their sex lives invariably spend a lot of time flirting, teasing, and playing. They don't wait until they're undressed. They trade sexy phone calls, full-body hugs in the hall, quick kisses that are more than a peck on the lips. Hot sex requires more than 0-to-60 intensity. You have to keep the embers glowing.

**PLAY WITH POSITIONS.** Even if you have a couple of favorites, take the initiative to do something new. Sex from behind instead of man on top. Interrupt intercourse to have oral sex rather than using your mouth only during foreplay. Try it standing, sitting, lying down. The great thing about sex is that there isn't a statute of limitations on play; you can experiment as often and in as many different ways as you like. As with anything else, it doesn't always work. You might find yourself doing more laughing than anything else. That's okay. That's great, actually. Intimacy means trusting each other enough to try just about anything. Don't worry about where you're going. Enjoy the journey.

## STEP 2: MAXIMIZE CONTROL

Maybe you're always hard when you want to be. Maybe you always come right when you want to. Maybe you always have the stamina to please your partner the way she wants to be pleased. Maybe you walk on water and can levitate a bottle of Bud from the refrigerator to the living room couch.

Unless you're a magician (or less than honest), sexual embarrassment is a fact of life. *Every* man has occasions when his body won't perform, when the heat of the moment gets doused with the cold water of a flagging erection or too-quick ejaculation. These and other sexual letdowns have little to do with your genetic makeup. Even when they're caused by physical problems—for example, buildups of cholesterol that inhibit bloodflow to the penis—they can almost always be minimized with a combination of exercise and lifestyle changes.

Did you know, for example, that you can dramatically improve your "holding" power with a series of exercises that takes just a couple of minutes a day? It's true. Specialists in sexual dysfunction clinics report that the vast majority of men who suffer from premature ejaculation can gain significant control by combining Kegel exercises with "squeeze" techniques that slow the rush to orgasm.

Want more motivation? Consider this: Men who practice these techniques—even men who already have good ejaculatory control—frequently report stronger and more intense orgasms. Along the way, some even develop the ability to have multiple orgasms.

## STEP 3: EXERCISE FOR BETTER SEX

Stretching, strength training, and cardiovascular workouts are the guts of the *Built for Sex* plan. Exercise increases the flow of energizing endorphins and adrenaline, body chemicals that make you feel strong, sexy, and confident. Guys who work out tend to have higher levels of testosterone, the male hormone you need for arousal as well as performance. Researchers at Cologne University Medical Centre in Germany even found that men who exercise have substantial increases of bloodflow to the penis—bloodflow that you need for erections.

We're not talking hard-core athletics. Men who work out *moderately* have increased sex drive and more predictable erections. In a landmark study, 78 sedentary, middle-age men did nothing more than aerobics four times a week. When researchers talked to them 9 months later, they learned that their frequency of sex had increased by nearly a third, and the frequency of orgasms had increased 26 percent.

And there are other exercise payoffs.

**INCREASED CONFIDENCE.** Men who exercise feel stronger and more energetic. They have more physical and mental confidence. They feel good in their own skins, and this goes a long way in the sexual realm.

**MORE ENERGY.** Even moderate levels of exercise—lifting a couple of times a week, for example, or taking daily walks—can stave off sex-killing fatigue. As a 54-year-old technical writer from Phoenix told us, *"I was sucking down pastries, chips, and sodas, and I was tired all the time. About a year ago, I made up my mind to get back to exercising, eating the right foods, and walking at lunch. I think my hormone levels must be up, because I want sex all the time."*

**LOOKING BETTER.** Lift weights a couple of times a week for a few months, and you're going to see the difference. You'll feel better when you look in the mirror. Your partner will enjoy looking at you. Now that's sexy.

**BETTER SEX**. The more you exercise, the more blood arrives in the penis. More blood means better erections. You'll be able to go longer without fatigue. And you'll *want* sex more than you did before.

You'll also be stronger and more limber—qualities you'll need if you even hope to try some of the more creative positions out there. Whether you want to get creative or stick with the tried and true, one simple exercise can kick it up a notch. Look at the "Position of Strength" section in chapter 6 for the specific exercise that strengthens the muscles you use for your favorite positions.

**LESS STRESS**. It's probably the main factor in low libido as well as erection problems. In fact, men who are stressed all the time find it almost impossible to have good sex because of destructive changes in body chemistry. Research has clearly shown that even lightweight exercise programs, such as occasional lifting, stretching, or aerobics, cause a dramatic drop in stress chemicals and an increase in sexual interest and activities.

**BETTER HEALTH**. It's hardly a secret that men who exercise are a lot less likely to get diabetes or hypertension, chronic and life-threatening diseases that are among the main causes of sexual problems.

Because exercise is so effective at improving appearance and physical and mental health, we've designed a total fitness plan that includes strength training, stretching, and cardiovascular workouts. You'll get stronger, in and out of bed. You'll have more sexual endurance, and you'll notice improvements in the muscles and joints that you need for good sex. We've even included exercises to improve ejaculatory control and increase the intensity of orgasms.

## THE *BUILT FOR SEX* PROMISE

Most of us are unconscious when it comes to our eating, exercise, and sexual habits. We do all sorts of things without really thinking about them. Many of these habits, unfortunately, drag us down rather than build us up. Do you have sex now as much as you did in your randy 20s? Probably not. If you're like most of us, the accrual of responsibilities and stress—job, family, money worries, and fatigue—has gradually eroded your lust for adventure and passion. You haven't given up sex, not by a long shot. You still want to exercise and look good. But do you think about it as much as you used to? Probably not.

You need to take the time to really tune into your life. Get a better sense of how you exercise. How you feel when you make love. If you're not entirely satisfied with what you see after a little bit of soul-searching—and it's doubtful that anyone is—it's time to add a couple of new habits and, sure, subtract a couple of the bad ones.

We understand that no man is going to turn his whole life upside down, even for the promise of more and better sex. Well, you don't have to. If you do nothing more than follow the steps in *any one* of the *Built for Sex* programs—technique adjustments, sexual control, strength training, and more—you're going to notice dramatic changes in how you feel and perform. You'll be a better lover. You'll achieve ejaculatory and erection control that you didn't have before. You'll please your partner more. You'll feel better about your body, your health, and your life.

The biggest challenge, one that's harder than changing your eating habits or contorting your limbs in highly erotic but unfamiliar ways, is to change the way you talk to yourself. Maybe you don't talk aloud, but if you're a man, you do talk to yourself, like cartoon characters who have an angel perched on one shoulder and a devil on the other. Unfortunately, the devil often gives the angel the boot. Not only does he tempt us into sin ("Hey, you're already overweight, what's another slice of cheesecake?"), he has an even more subtle tool for undercutting your self-confidence. Call it the "if . . . then" way of thinking. "If you can just lose 20 pounds," the devil tells you, "then you'll feel great and have better sex."

That kind of thinking gets you nowhere because the rewards are always delayed. If you're really going to get motivated, you have to learn to appreciate who you are and where you are in your life. Don't start this plan because you're dissatisfied with where you are now. Start it because you know you deserve the best life has to offer, and there's no better time to start than now.

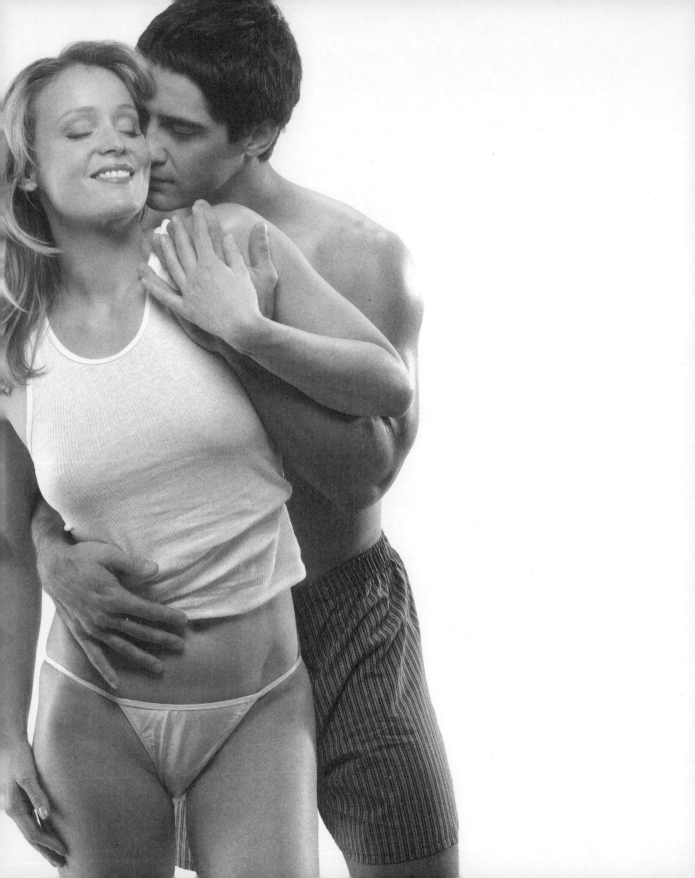

# PART 1

# HONE YOUR TECHNIQUE

# CHAPTER 1

# BETTER SEX TECHNIQUE: A REFRESHER COURSE

**ONCE YOU STRIP AWAY THE SUBTLE VARIATIONS, THERE ARE SIX BASIC POSITIONS FOR HAVING SEX:** man on top, woman on top, side by side, sitting, standing, and rear entry. Each has advantages and disadvantages, such as deeper penetration, more body-to-body contact, or ease of performing when you're tired. But why make it complicated? Most couples choose a certain sexual position, or a variety of them, for no other reason than they like them—although physical changes (such as her pregnancy or your back pain) may shift your preferences one way or another.

You're already familiar with the basic positions (illustrated over the next 32 pages), but it might be useful to know what makes each one unique—in terms of comfort, what gets stimulated, how men and women respond, and so on. You'll also discover a few variations that you may want to try.

## POSITION #1: MAN ON TOP

It's probably the most popular sexual position in this country because it allows face-to-face intimacy and full-body contact and permits deep thrusts and full penetration. It's comfortable for the woman because she can lie on her back, with or without a pillow to change the angle; men like it because they can control the timing and penetration.

There are a few drawbacks, however. This "missionary position" can be too arousing for men in some cases, causing too-quick ejaculation. A small woman with a bulky partner may find his weight uncomfortable unless he takes care to support his weight on his arms. From a man's point of view, it can be tiring because he's doing most of the heavy lifting.

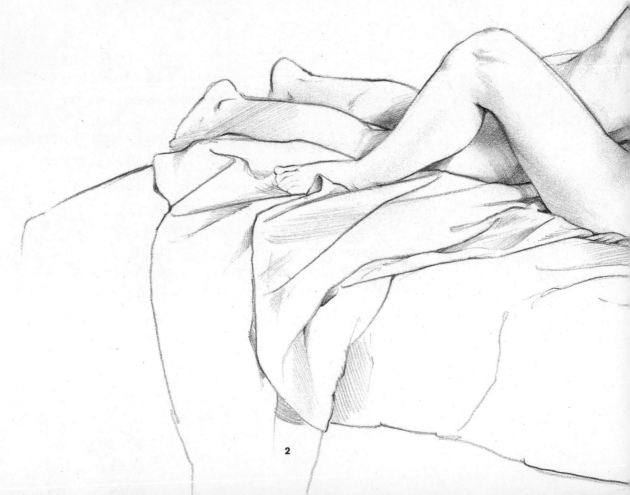

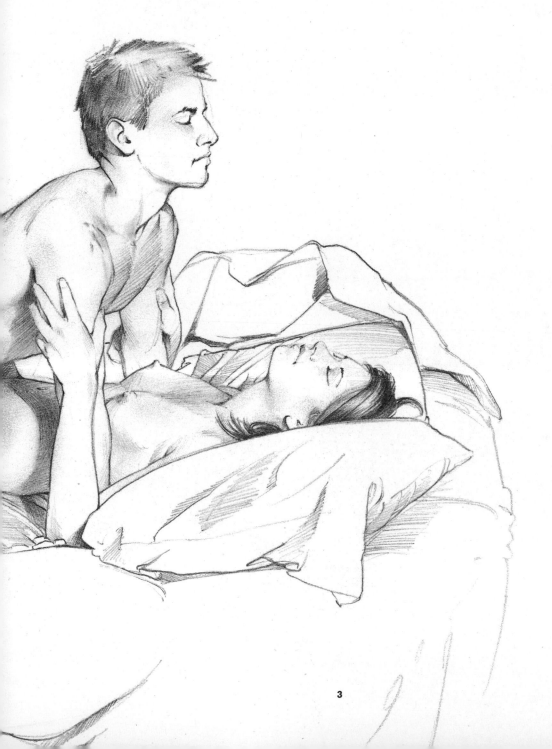

**MAN ON TOP (VARIATION)**

The woman can wrap her legs around your waist or neck or rest them on your shoulders. You can raise her legs by putting your forearms under her knees.

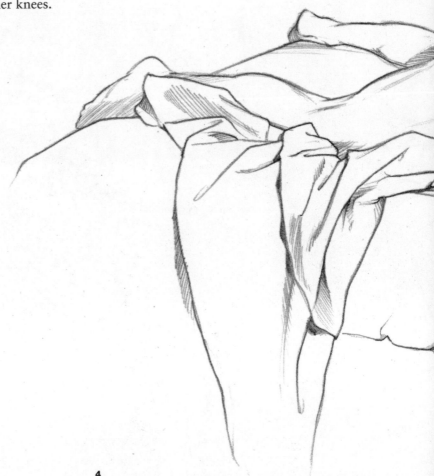

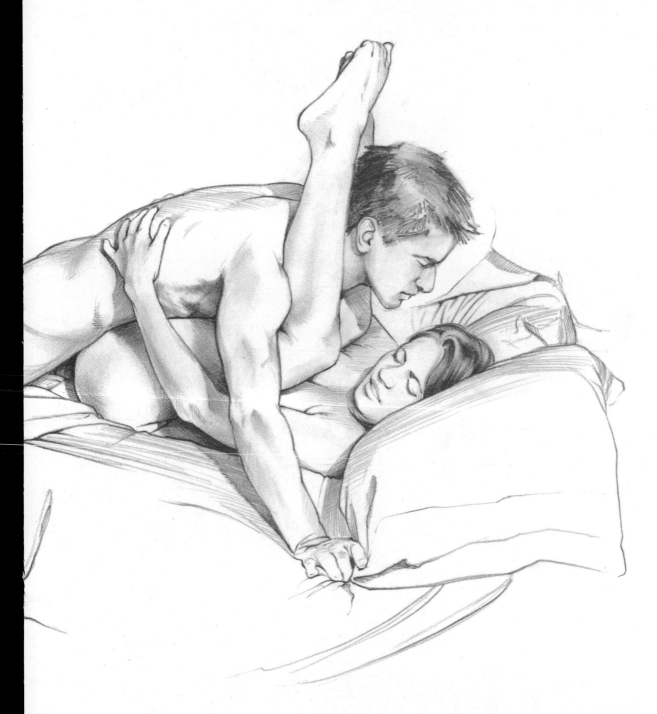

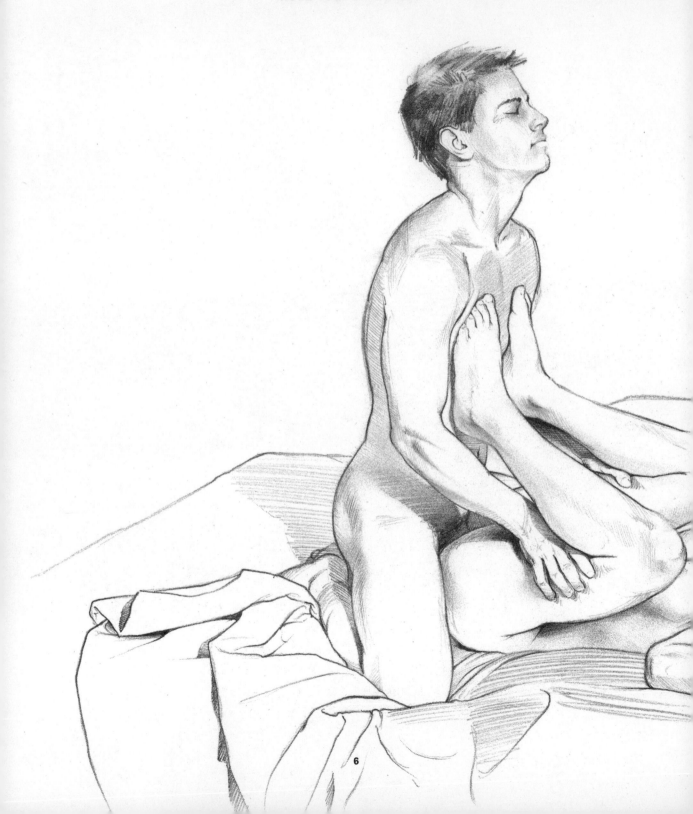

**MAN ON TOP (VARIATION)**

The woman can pull her knees to her chest and put her feet flat against your chest.

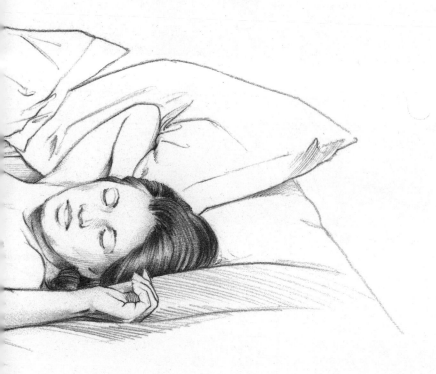

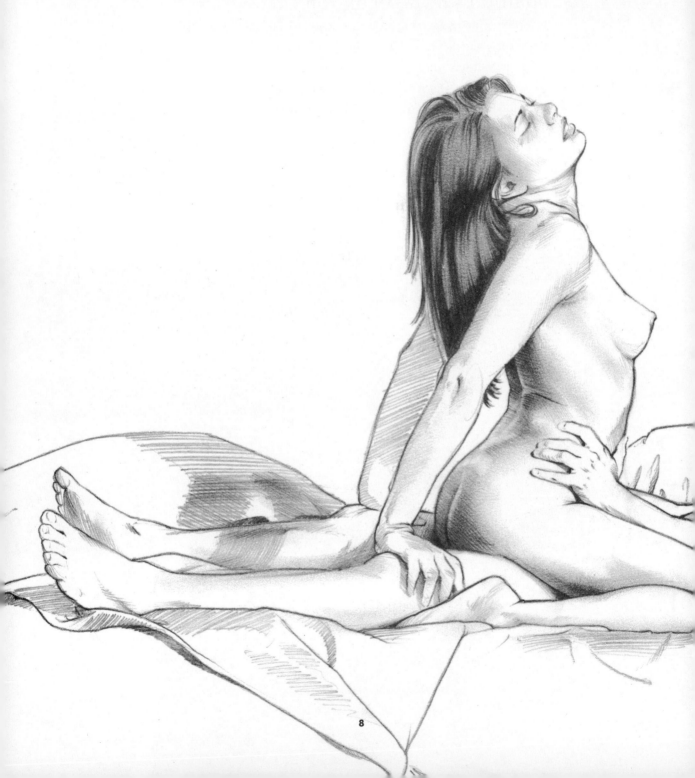

## POSITION #2: WOMAN ON TOP

It's second in popularity only to the missionary position. The woman straddles your pelvis and raises and lowers herself on your penis. Like the man-on-top position, it allows you to kiss and make eye contact. The woman controls the pace as well as the angle of penetration, and she can stimulate her clitoris while you're making love.

Most men find this position visually as well as physically stimulating. You can watch your partner as she moves up and down, and your hands are free to caress her face, breasts, or buttocks. The depth of penetration equals that of the man-on-top position, which is pleasurable for both partners.

The drawbacks are the reverse of man on top. In this position, the woman rather than the man may find herself getting tired. Also, women who are self-conscious about their bodies may be somewhat uncomfortable with having them in full view.

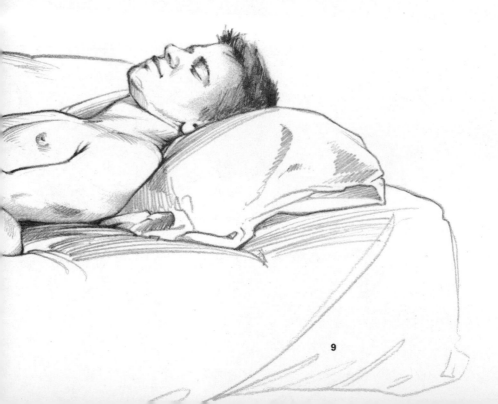

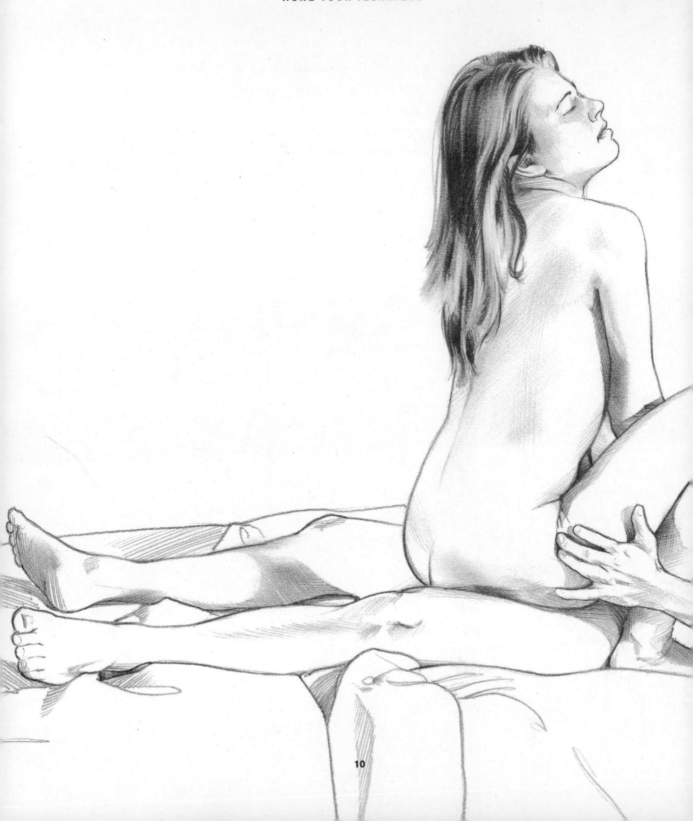

### WOMAN ON TOP (VARIATION)

The woman can lean forward to rest her hands on the bed in front of her or on your chest.

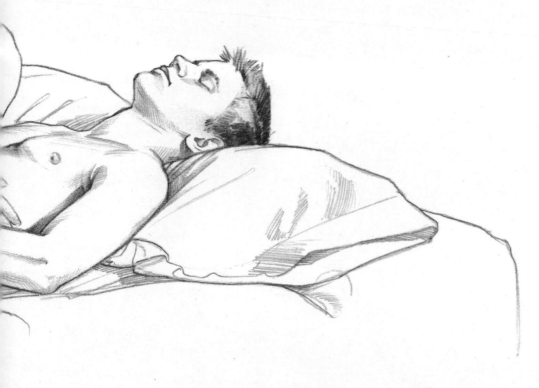

**WOMAN ON TOP (VARIATION)**

The woman can turn around so
she's facing your feet.

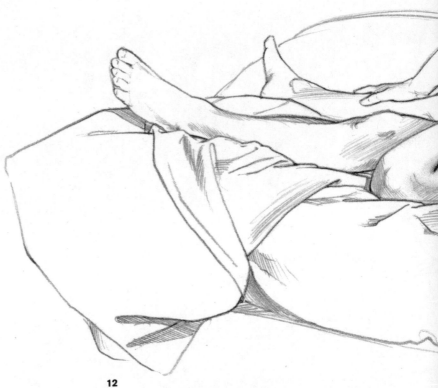

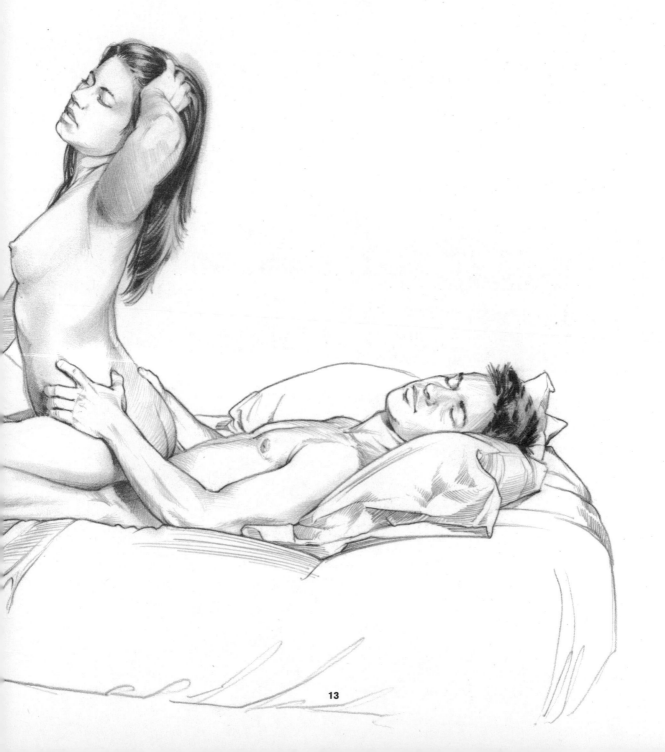

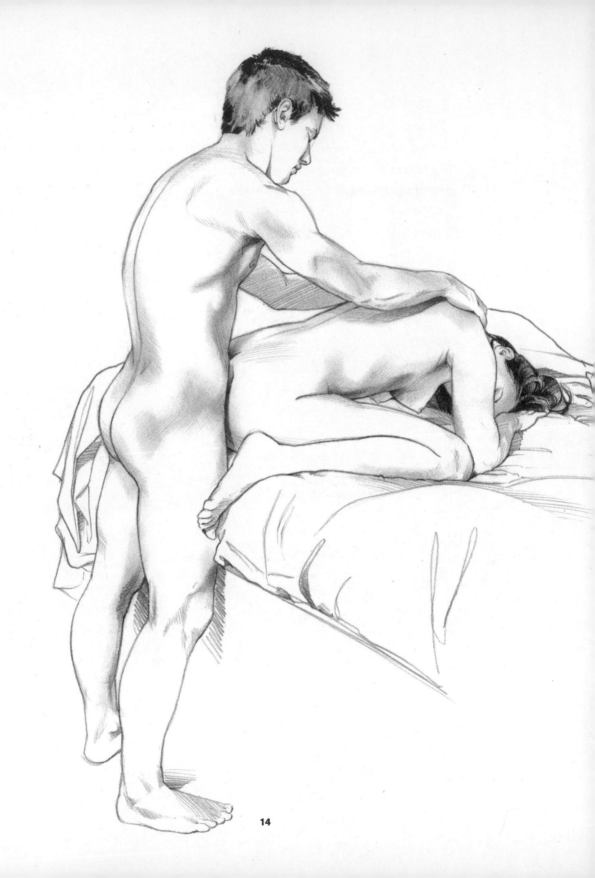

14

## POSITION #3: REAR ENTRY

The woman gets on her knees and elbows while you enter her from behind. Many women say that this is the best position for stimulating the G-spot. It also gives her visual imagination full play; when you're out of sight, she can fill her mind with whatever fantasies she likes.

Men often enjoy this position because it gives them a sense of power and dominance, while at the same time allowing deep and vigorous thrusting. They can also reach around and touch the woman's breasts or clitoris or enjoy it while she touches herself.

The rear-entry position is less intimate than other positions, however, and some women don't like to be "taken" in the position disparagingly known as doggie style.

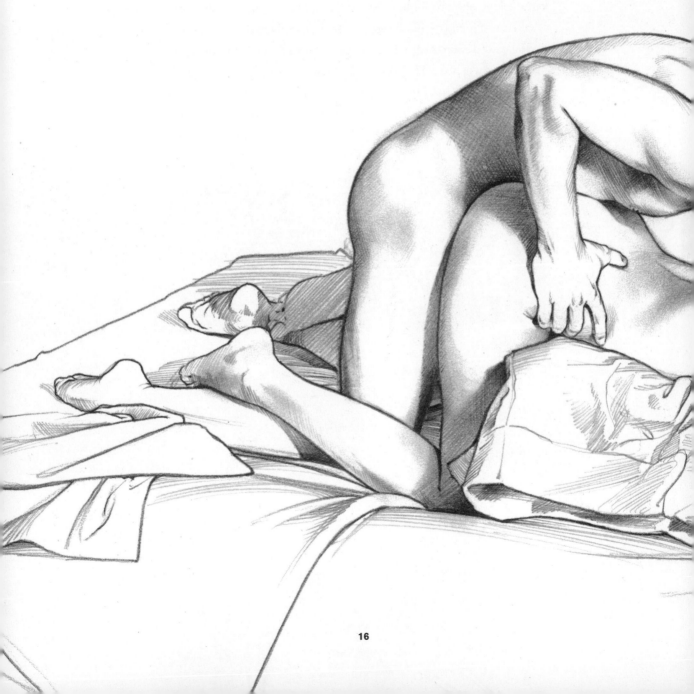

**REAR ENTRY (VARIATION)**
The woman can lie on her stomach with her bottom elevated.

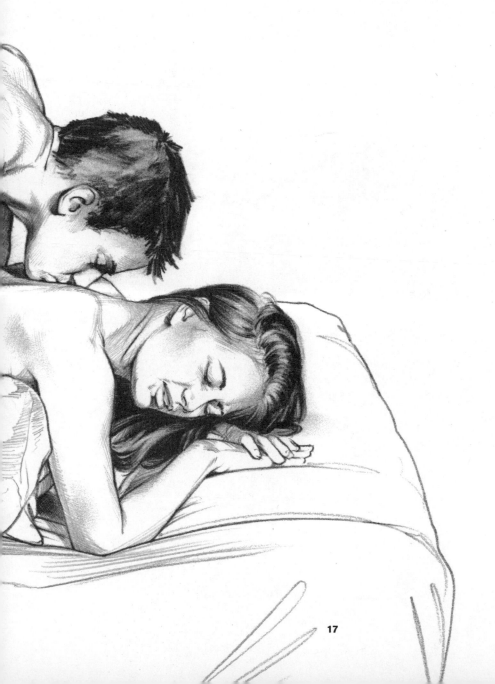

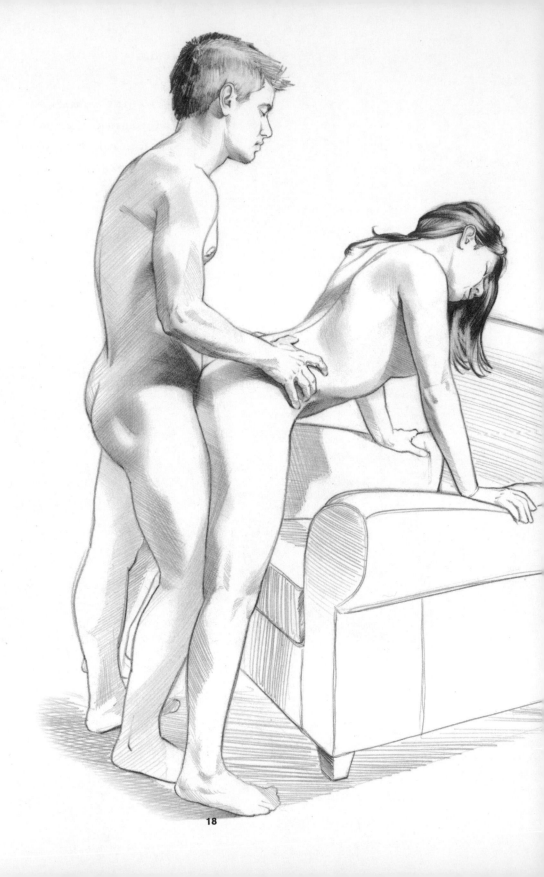

18

**REAR ENTRY (VARIATION)**

The woman can stand while bending over and holding a chair or a nightstand for support.

## POSITION #4: SIDE BY SIDE

You and your partner face each other while lying on your sides. It's a good position when you're both a little tired. It's also a comfortable position if you happen to have back pain or the woman is pregnant. Side-by-side sex tends to be languorous and slow. It's easy for both partners to touch each other, and since you don't achieve deep penetration, ejaculation is often delayed.

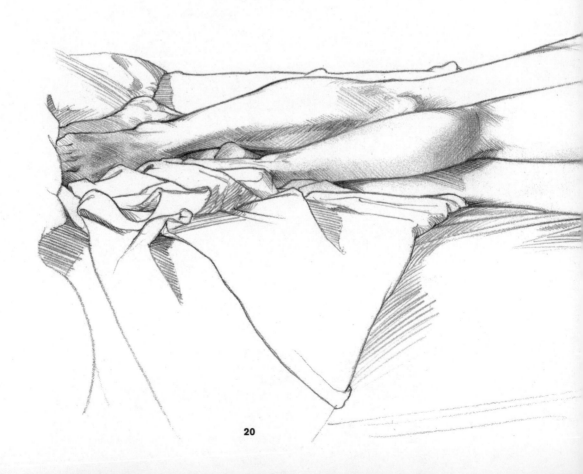

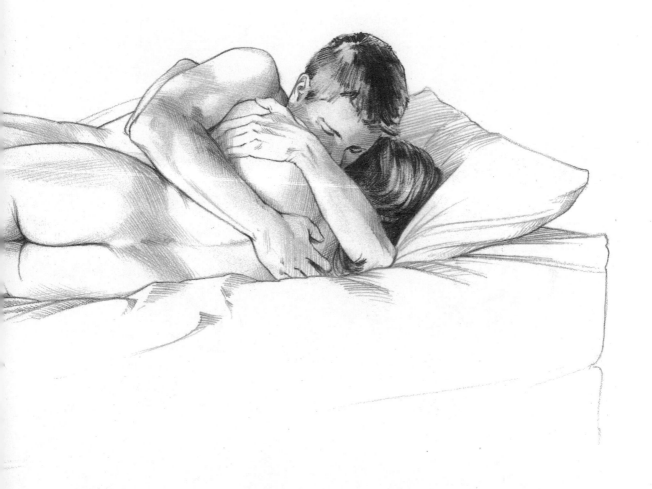

**SIDE BY SIDE (VARIATION)**

You can "spoon" together, with the woman's backside nestled against you.

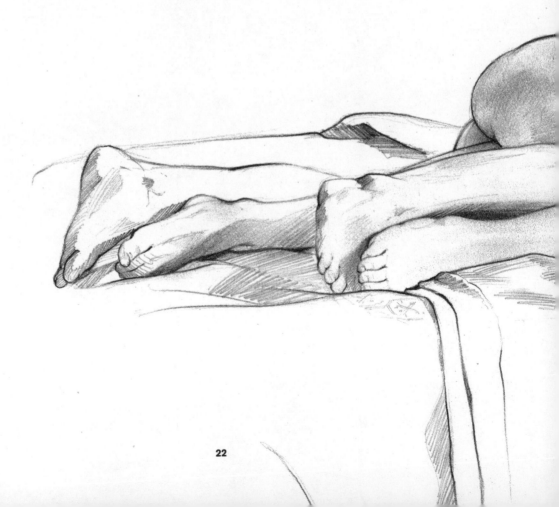

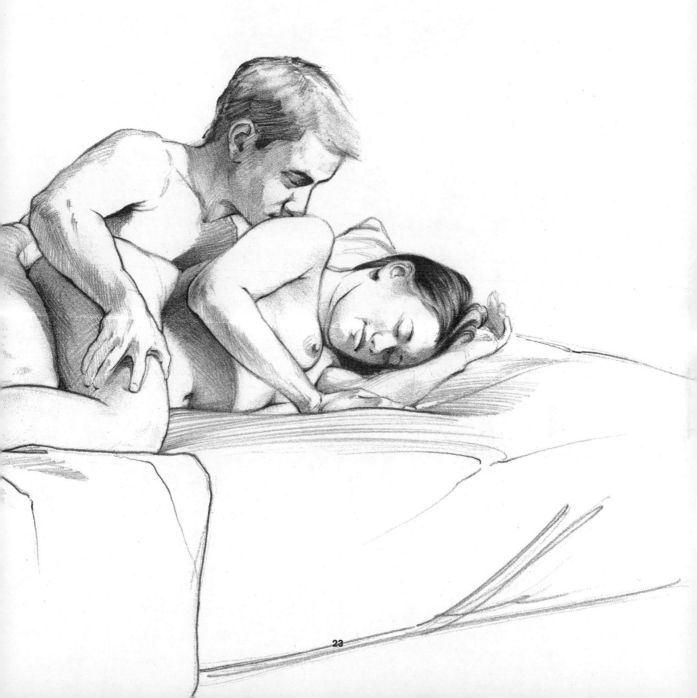

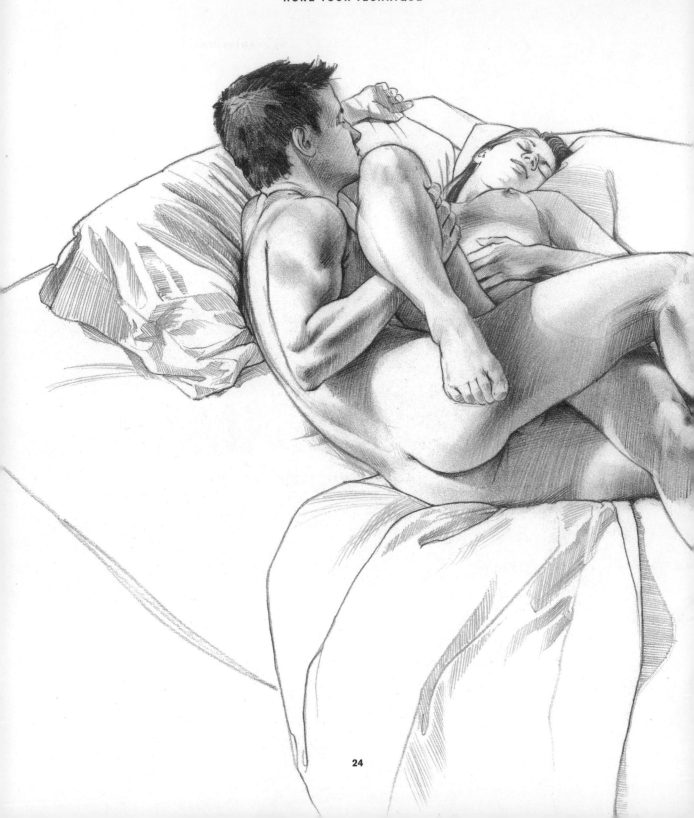

### SIDE BY SIDE (VARIATION)

You can lie on your side while the woman lies on her back, one leg between your thighs and the other leg on top.

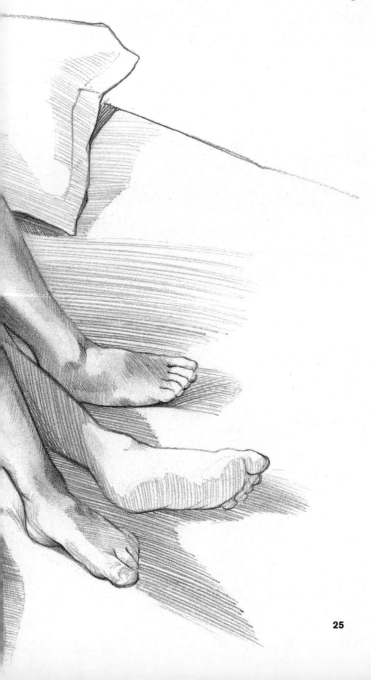

## POSITION #5: SITTING

You sit on the bed while your partner sits on your lap in a face-to-face position. It's a very intimate position that permits a lot of kissing and touching. It's visually stimulating because you can fully see what your partner is doing.

Having sex while sitting is physically taxing. You have to have strong abdominal muscles to hold yourself upright. Penetration can be fairly deep, but you can't move quickly in this position.

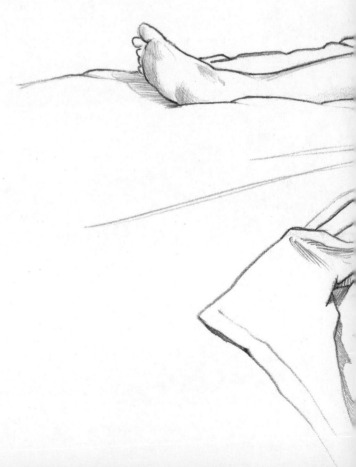

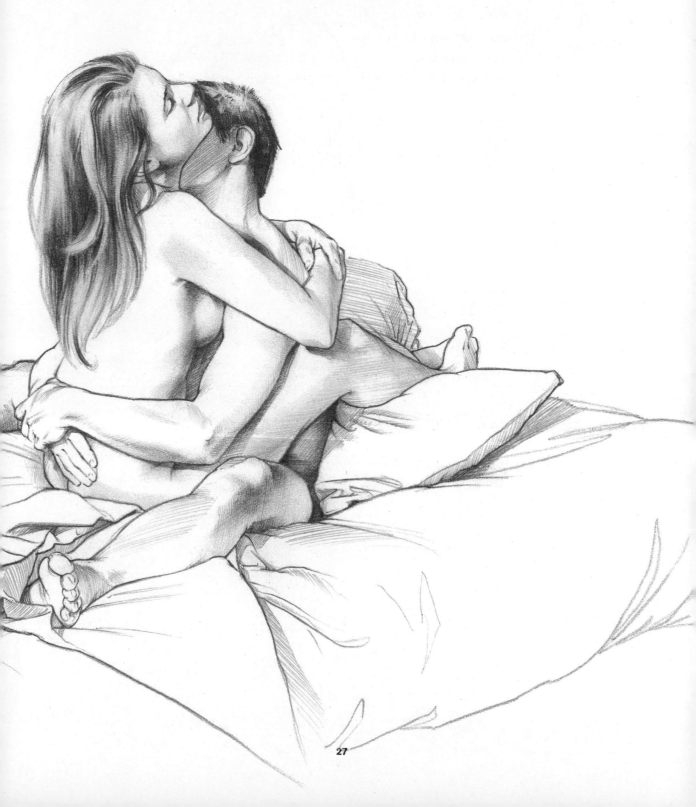

### SITTING (VARIATION)

The woman can turn so that her back is against your chest.

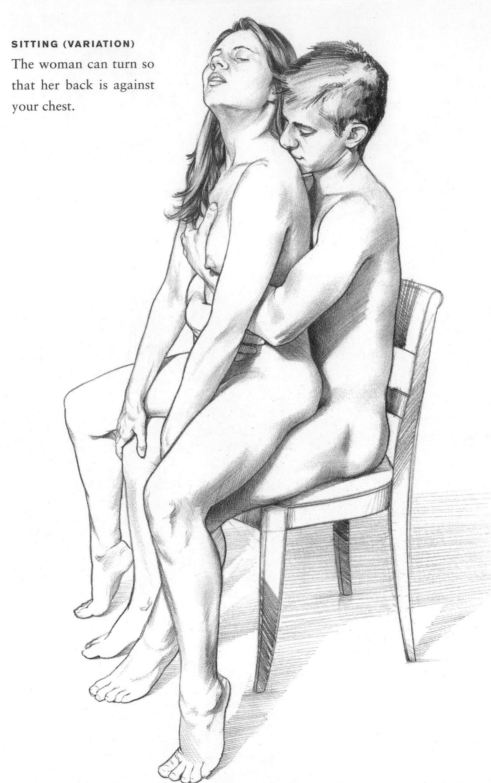

## SITTING (VARIATION)

The woman can straddle you face to face in a chair, then lean all the way back to rest her head on a pillow on the floor.

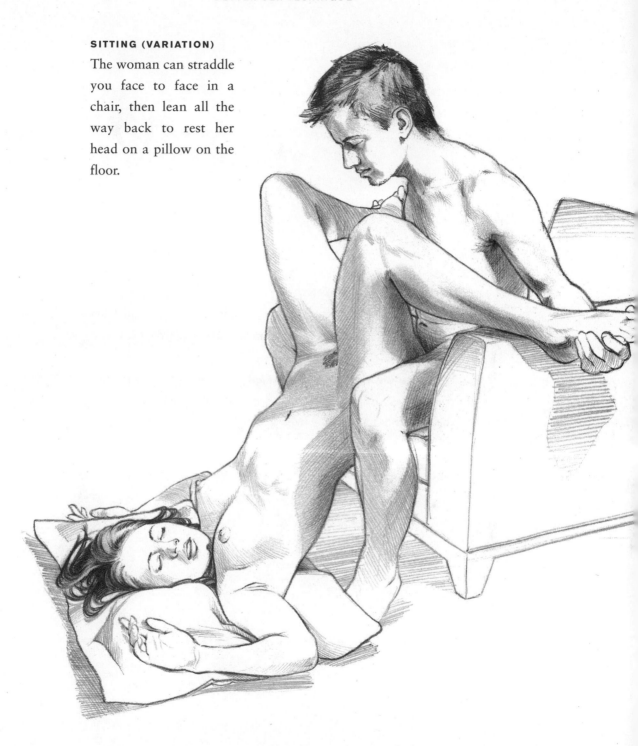

## POSITION #6: STANDING

It's a good position for spontaneous lovemaking—quickies, in other words. You can enter the woman from the rear while she leans forward slightly.

This position requires more strength and dexterity than most other sexual positions. Don't try it if you have a bad back, or if your partner is too heavy to maneuver safely.

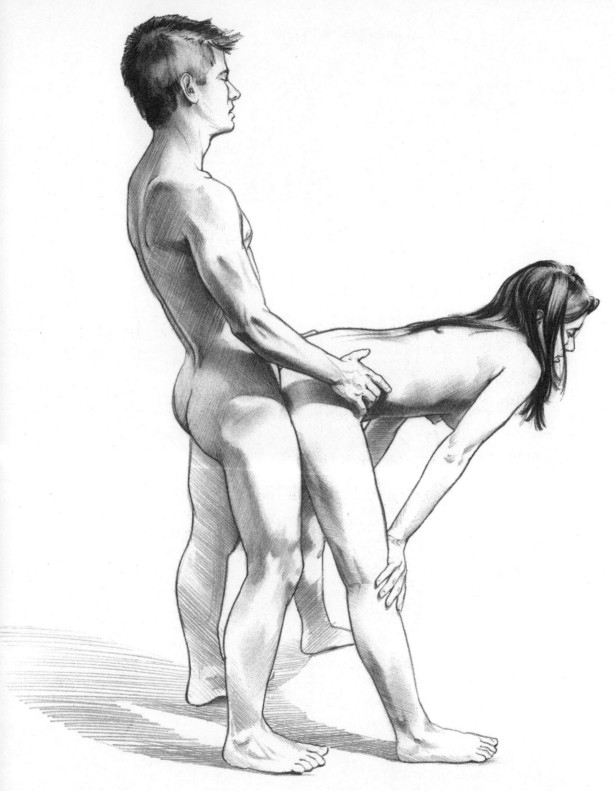

31

### STANDING (VARIATION)

You can lift the woman with your arms, facing you, and hold her thighs while moving her up and down.

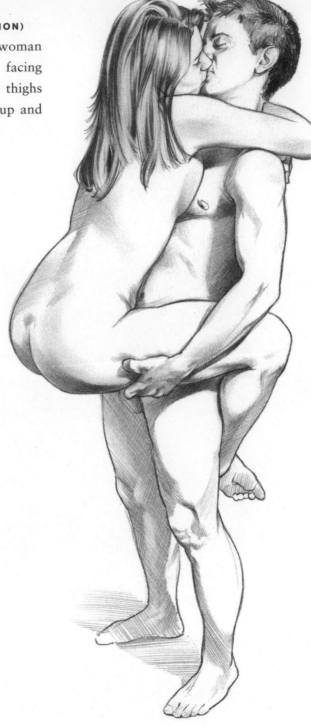

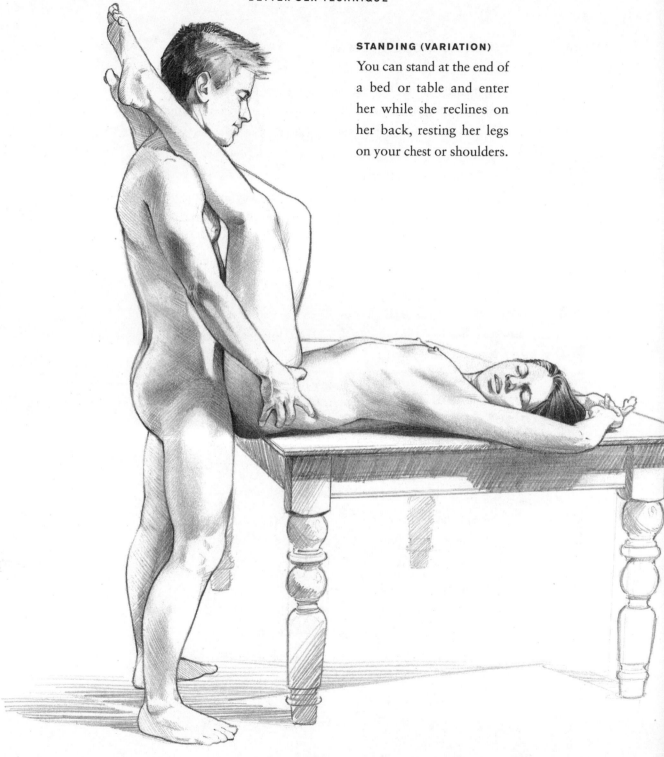

## STANDING (VARIATION)

You can stand at the end of a bed or table and enter her while she reclines on her back, resting her legs on your chest or shoulders.

## CREATIVE COUPLING

No matter how much you and your partner enjoy the old favorites, you might want to have some fun now and then and experiment with something totally new. It's true that there is only a handful of core positions, but each of these has almost infinite variations.

One caveat: Many of these positions take practice. If you have a mental image of porn-star dexterity and polish, you're going to be disappointed. You won't have any trouble mastering these positions, but it's going to take practice. Don't take yourself too seriously; enjoy the trying. *"Orgasms are great, but they also signal the temporary end of the fun,"* a 48-year-old firefighter told us. *"We focus more on the journey than the arrival."*

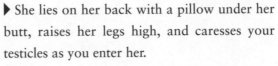

**"Sex is like snow: You never know how many inches you're going to get or how long it will last."**
**—ANONYMOUS**

▶ She lies on her back with a pillow under her butt, raises her legs high, and caresses your testicles as you enter her.

▶ She lies on her back with a pillow under her butt, legs open. You kneel between her thighs while sitting back on your ankles. Grip her thighs and pull her toward you. She can touch her clitoris while making love, and you can massage her breasts and arms.

▶ She lies on the bed or couch with her legs over the edge and her feet on the floor. You kneel and enter her without getting off your knees.

▶ Lie on your back with your legs spread at the knees. She straddles your thighs, feet resting on the bed and supporting herself with her hands, and rocks vigorously.

▶ Lie on your back with your legs apart. She straddles you, then lowers her chest to yours. She closes her thighs and clamps your penis firmly inside.

▶ Lie on your back while she straddles you. Once you're inside, sit up together and wrap your arms around each other. Sit perfectly still as your sexual energy rises. Then move gently back and forth.

▶ She lies facedown while you kneel between her legs. Pull her close and lift her buttocks for easier entry and movement.

▶ Sit on a chair while she lowers herself onto your lap, back facing you. Using her arms and legs for support, she raises and lowers herself, setting the pace and depth of penetration.

▶ She stands on a step to bring her height closer to yours, and you enter her while standing.

▶ Stand facing one another. Raise one of her legs with your hands and enter her. She supports herself with the other leg while wrapping her arms around you.

# CHAPTER 2

# NEXT-LEVEL TECHNIQUES

**AS A MAN, YOU'RE HARDWIRED FOR SEXUAL VARIETY. AND THAT'S NOT JUST YOUR PENIS TALKING. IT'S YOUR BRAIN.** Our biological bartender, Mother Nature, serves up a carnal cocktail of hormones that keeps you buzzing so you seek out sexual adventures that ultimately populate the planet.

It starts when you're single. Testosterone urges you out to bars and beaches to scout for potential mates. Once you find one, you're rewarded with a rush of amphetamine-like hormones, such as dopamine, that sends you on a hedonistic high of nonstop sex drive. You'll do it anytime, anywhere—atop the dryer, on the kitchen floor, in the garage. As time marches on with the same mate, however, that natural rush is replaced with a more mellow high from brain chemicals like vasopressin and oxytocin that calm you down enough to hold a job and raise a family. These so-called attachment chemicals leave you feeling relaxed, satisfied—and frankly, a little bored.

The key to fanning the flames is either finding a new woman (generally not an option) or pulling a fast one on Mother Nature. New positions, toys, games, and even fantasy play can make you see your partner in a whole new way—literally—by tricking your brain into responding with that feels-like-the-first-time rush. Don't take just our word for it. Women, too, need change to keep sexually charged. As a 33-year-old graphic artist from Atlanta told us. *"It's easy to get caught up in a sex routine when you've been with the same person for awhile. To keep your sex life active, you need an open mind and adventurous spirit. I enjoy being able to laugh as much as I moan (and I do both fairly loudly) during sex because we're experimenting and having fun."*

## 9 POSITIONS YOU DIDN'T LEARN IN SEX ED

Famed sex researcher Alfred Kinsey, PhD, once estimated that the missionary position was the only position used by 70 percent of the adult population. Don't tell that to the women we surveyed for this book, who unanimously rated trying new sexual positions as "very important." We flipped through ancient manuals like the *Kama Sutra* as well as some popular Web sites to bring you an arsenal of innovative, sometimes athletic, positions for sex play that should keep the fun in your bedroom for years to come.

A word to the wise: These positions may require some work (and maybe a few failed attempts) to achieve, but the payoff may be a new favorite. Says one 41-year-old Pittsburgh bartender, *"When we first started playing with new positions, it seemed more like acrobatics than sex. But a couple of times we hit upon something really, really good. That's when all the ones that didn't work out were definitely worth the effort."*

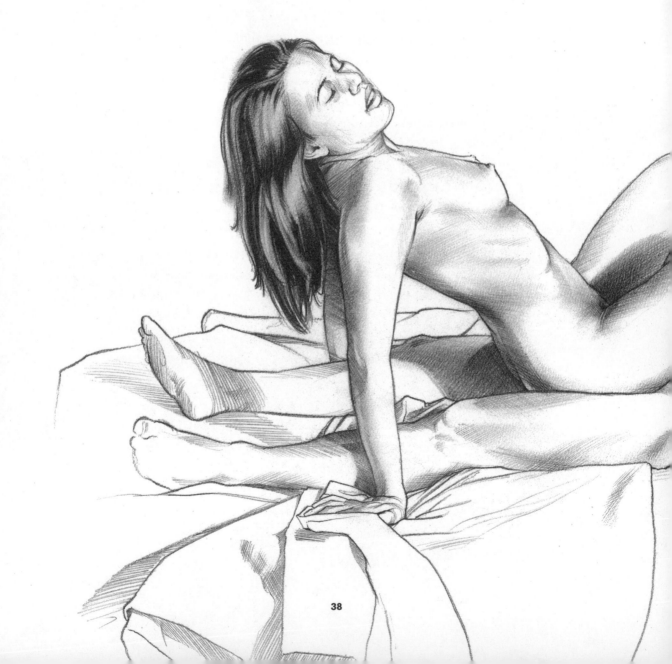

## HEAD OVER HEELS

This unconventional position turns traditional sex on its head. You lie on your back with your legs slightly bent and apart. She straddles you in the classic woman-on-top position and then lies all the way back, so her feet are next to your head and her head is down by your feet. She does most of the "thrusting" by sliding back and forth along your penis.

If your penis doesn't bend that way comfortably, you can make this position more accessible by bending your knees to let her rest her back on your thighs in more of a reclining position.

*Why she likes it:* With her feet up by your head, you can indulge her in some decadent foot rubbing and toe sucking during intercourse.

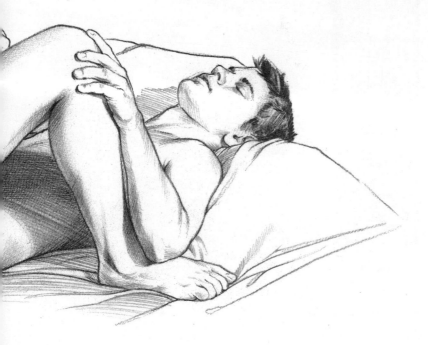

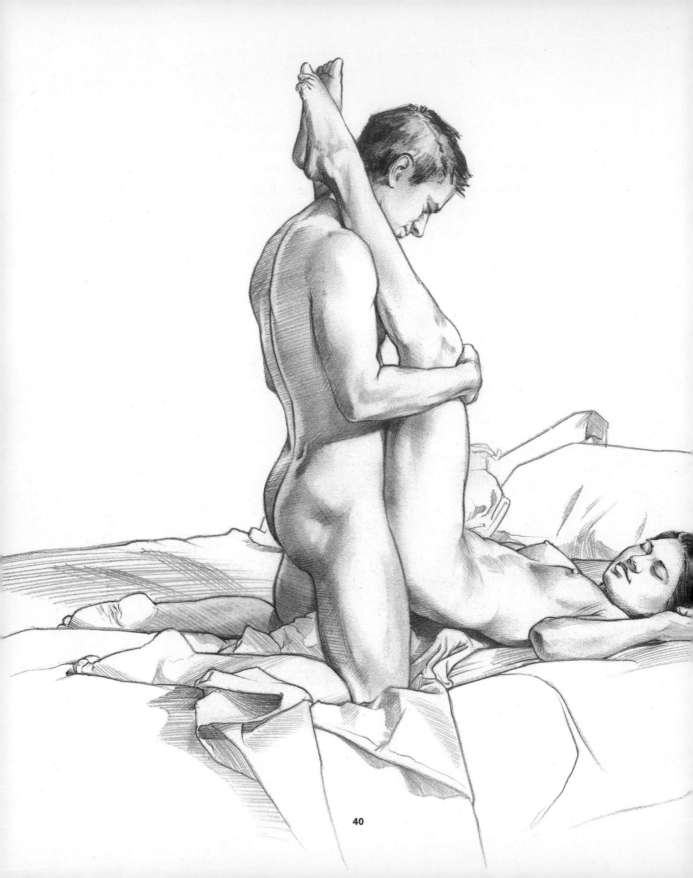

40

## SKIN THE CAT

In this inverted position, your partner lies flat on her back; you kneel between her knees and lift her legs up and over your shoulders, so only her head and shoulders remain on the bed, and she is suspended with her calves resting on either side of your neck. You then slide your penis downward into her.

You can grasp her thighs and pull her toward you rhythmically to assist in thrusting. You also can slide your hands down and caress her clitoris for added pleasure. Though thrusting is easy from the kneeling position, men with steeply angled erections may find the downward motion of this position difficult.

*Why she likes it:* Being upside down gives her a giddy head rush and feeling of weightlessness during intercourse and allows her to caress her breasts.

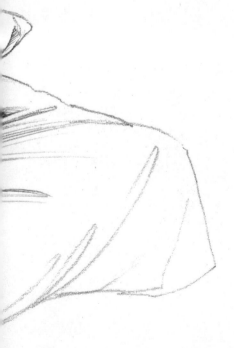

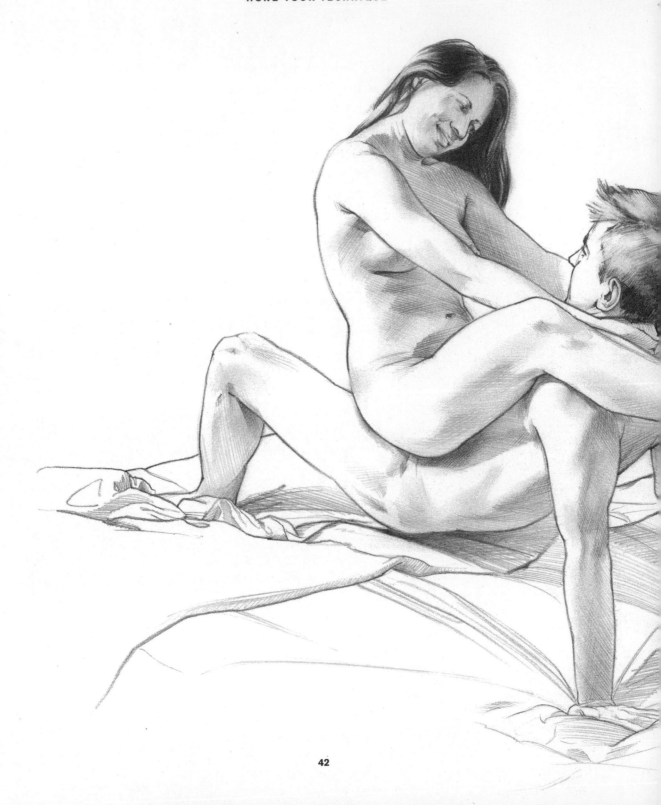

## THE HONEYBEE

This part-sitting, part-reclining position allows maximum penetration and visual stimulation, though it requires a fair amount of strength and flexibility from both of you. You sit, leaning back with your hands on the bed behind your back for support. She straddles your penis, placing both legs over your shoulders and holding on to either side of your neck with her hands. To thrust, you press your thighs together, lifting her up, then open them wide, letting her slide back down, repeating so your legs make a "fluttering" motion.

The tricky part is maintaining insertion while getting into position. If she's fairly flexible, you may want to let her straddle you in the classic woman-on-top position first, then shift to place her legs over your shoulders. Otherwise, assume the position without inserting; then you can lean back and gently guide your penis into her.

*Why she likes it:* Her vaginal wall is angled upward, allowing for more intense G-spot stimulation with every thrust.

## GAME DAY

This is a perfect position for spontaneous Sunday-afternoon sex when your favorite team is winning. You sit on a couch or cushioned armchair. She straddles you, placing her legs up and over the back or sides of the couch or chair. She can place her hands on your shoulders or place them on your knees behind her.

This position allows for a lot of variety. You can wrap your arms around each other for increased face-to-face and skin-on-skin intimacy, or she can lie all the way back and simply enjoy the ride.

*Why she likes it:* The seated pelvic contact here gives her extra clitoral stimulation with every thrust. Plus, you have easy access to kiss her breasts and caress her body.

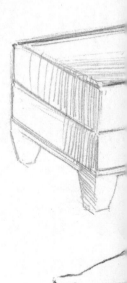

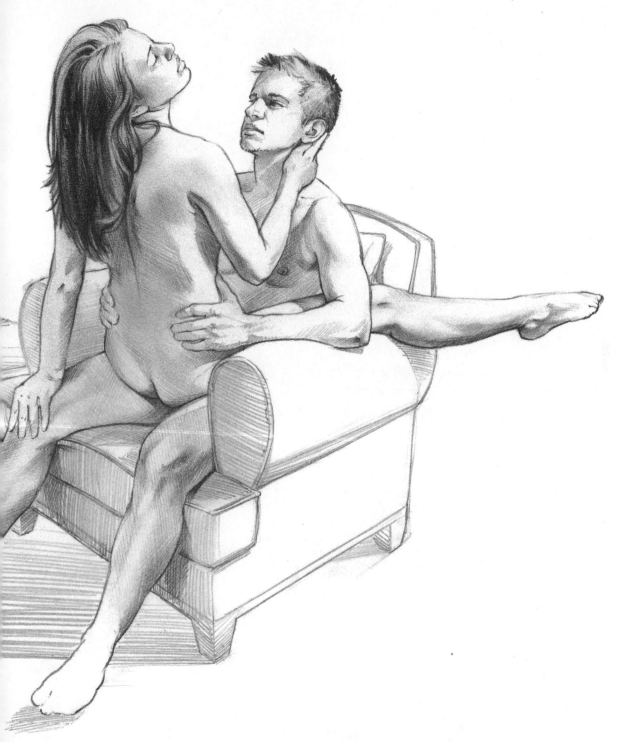

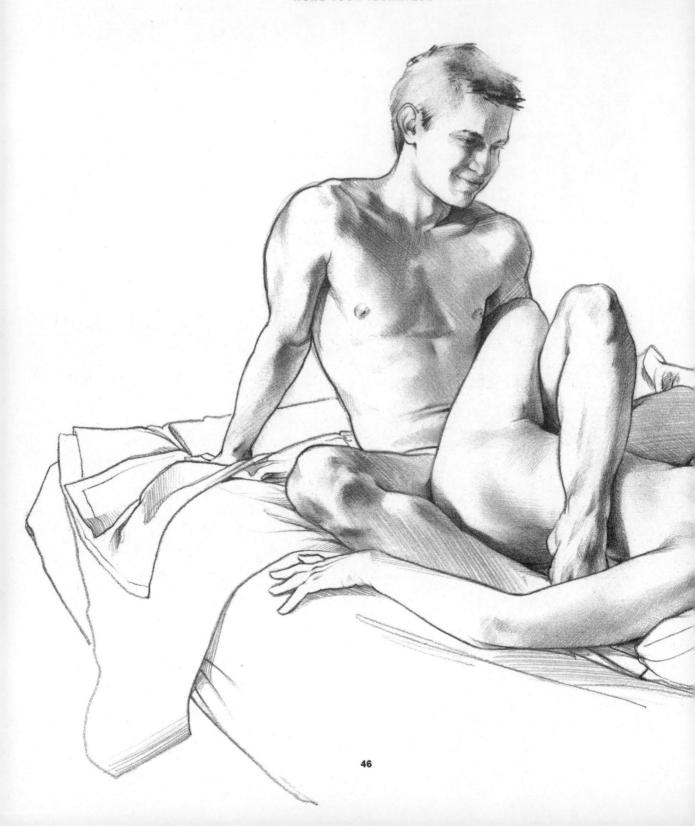

## SCISSORS

Fun sex is a little like spirited grappling, and this move is reminiscent of something you might see in the WWF—only you both win. She lies back on the bed with her legs bent and thighs apart. You sit between her knees and place your right leg between her thighs so your right foot is resting by her ribs under her left arm. Grasp her left leg and bring it across your body, holding it under your left arm. Slide into her, then place your hands behind you on the bed for thrusting support. This position looks harder to achieve than it actually is, though it does require a fair amount of penile flexibility.

*Why she likes it:* Her clitoris will get extra stimulation as it rubs against your inner thigh during thrusting.

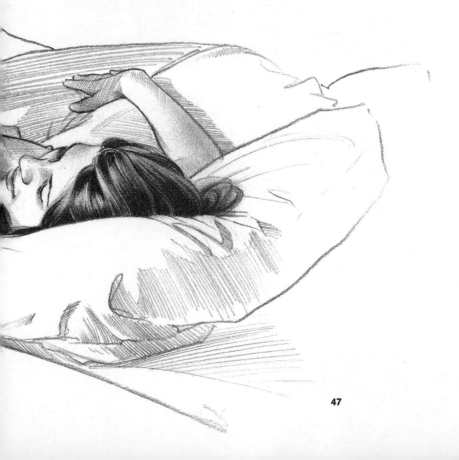

## BLUE MOON

Like all good positions, this one begins sexy and gets hotter as it progresses. To begin, you lie face up on the bed as usual. She straddles you facing your feet. Once your penis is fully inserted, she bends all the way forward, so her breasts are resting on your thighs and her face is down by your shins. She also can extend her legs slightly to fully drape herself over you as you thrust in unison.

*Why she likes it:* She can rub her breasts against your legs. And you can increase her pleasure by rubbing her buttocks and caressing her labia as you slide in and out of her.

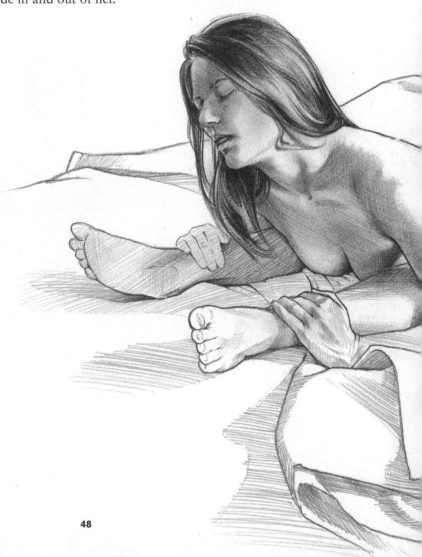

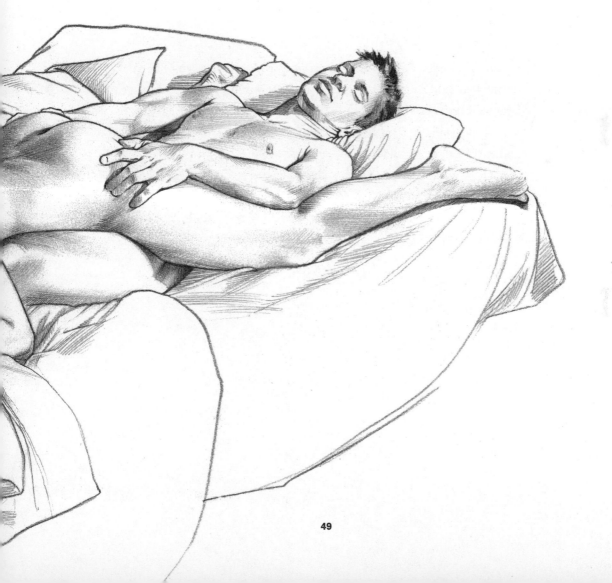

## ON BENDED KNEE

In this erotic take on the classic marriage proposal pose, you kneel on the bed, and she kneels down in front of you with her right leg bent so it drapes over your left leg and the lower part of her left leg extended behind her for balance and support. Hold onto her hips and enter her, thrusting as you normally would.

If she is a lot shorter than you, she may need to kneel on pillows to achieve this position.

*Why she likes it:* This position has romantic undertones and allows for lots of face-to-face intimacy, kissing, and caressing.

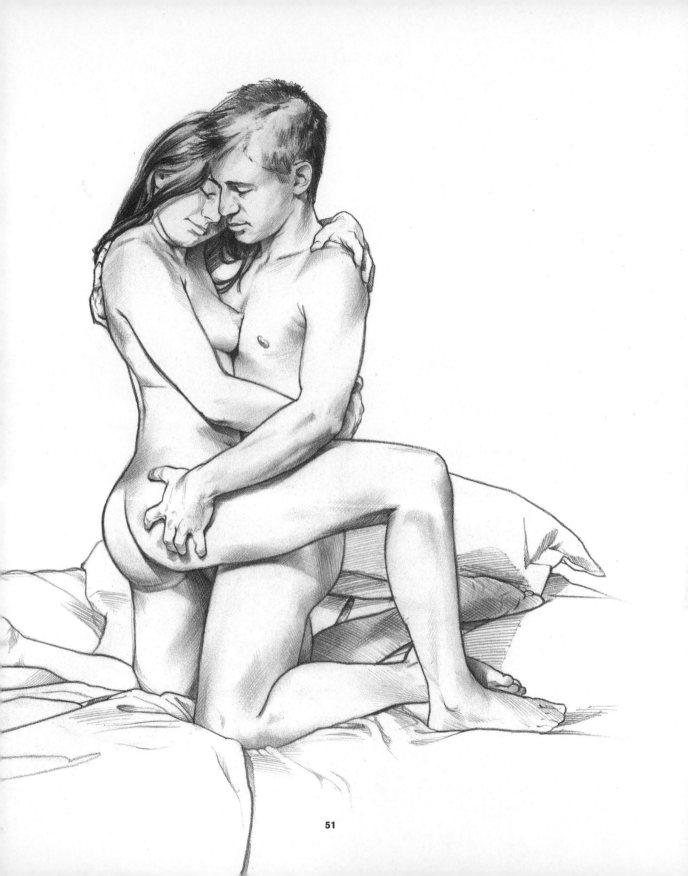

## THE WHEELBARROW

As the name implies, this position harkens back to the childhood game where you pick up someone's legs as if using a wheelbarrow. Only now it's a lot more fun. Have your partner lie facedown on a carpeted floor. Step between her feet, grasp her legs, and lift her lower body off the floor. As you lift, she should straighten her arms and support herself on her hands, so you can lift her vagina to you and slide your penis into her from behind.

*Why she likes it:* This variation of the rear-entry position tilts her pelvis so she feels more G-spot stimulation with every thrust.

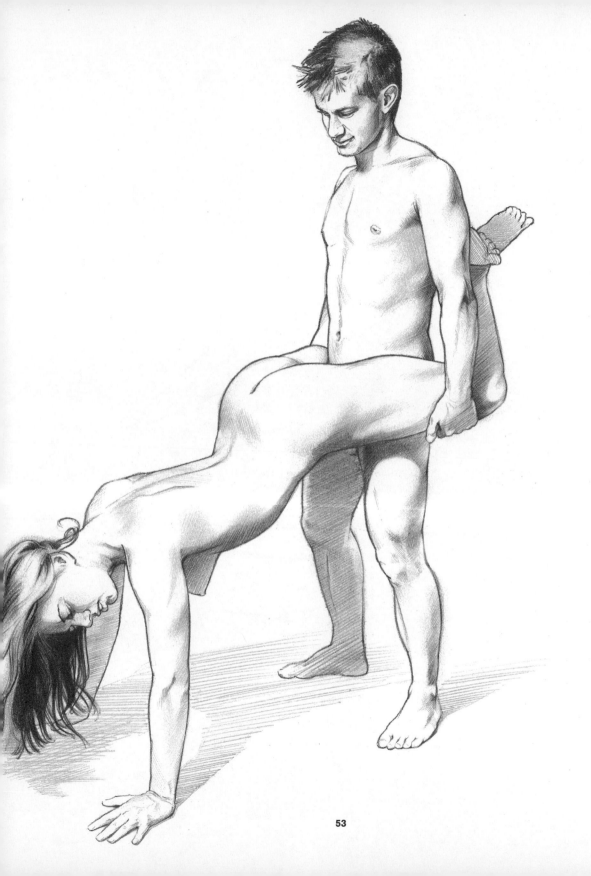

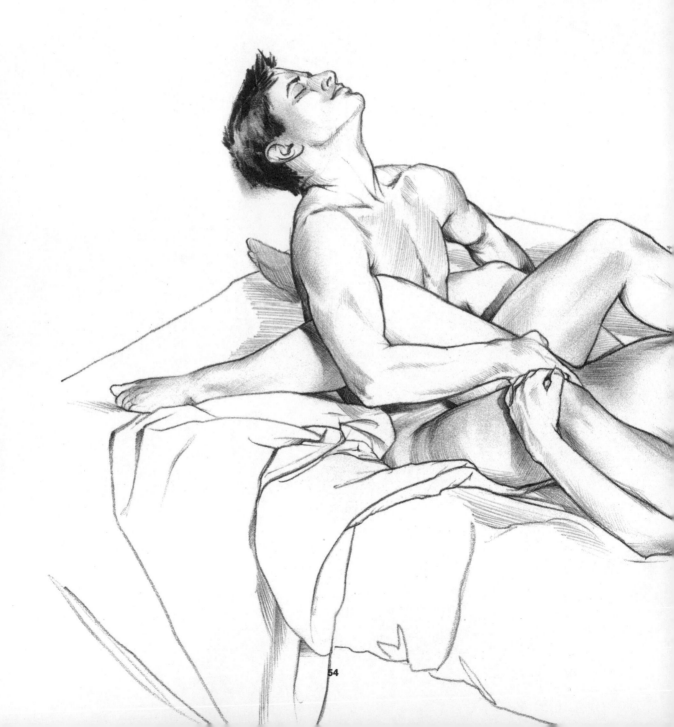

## THE PRETZEL

In this twisty-turny position, you recline with your right leg extended and your left leg bent. Your thighs should be apart and your torso should be off the bed about 45 degrees. She lies between your legs with her head on the bed by your right foot, weaving her right leg under your left and draping her left leg over your right as you enter her. She wraps her left arm around your right thigh, and you hold onto her waist for thrusting leverage.

*Why she likes it:* This pretzel position gives her easy access to massage her clitoris at a pressure she enjoys while fully reclined and comfortable.

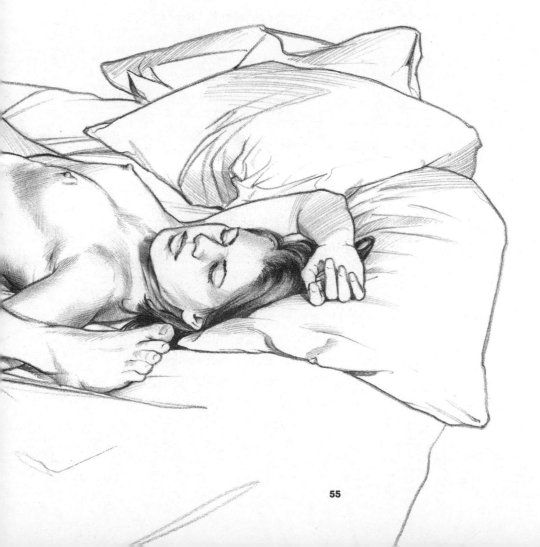

## TOYS FOR TWO

Sexual aids have been used around the globe for more than a thousand years. Back in the day, they were mostly considered male-replacement apparatus. The Greek *olisbos* and Italian *diletto* were designed to give solace to lonely women whose husbands were out fighting or foraging. In the Victorian era, doctors actually invented the first vibrator, used to treat "female hysteria," literally "suffering of the uterus." Today, toys are used as much, if not more, for couple fun as for solitary pleasure—and vibrators seem to be the toy of choice. "*A vibrator is a fun way to mix things up during sex,*" says a 38-year-old software engineer from Eatontown, New Jersey. "*It also helps me know my body better, which is helpful for both of us.*" Some women especially like to use their toys on their partners. Said one 44-year-old nurse from Jacksonville, Florida, "*Sex toys make it easier to see how your handiwork is pleasing your partner. That's a big turn on.*"

The take-home lesson: If you're interested, talk to your partner. Surf women-friendly Web sites like www.goodvibes.com or www.babeland.com and pick out a toy for each of you. Here's a primer to get you started.

**VIBRATORS**. These popular toys come in all shapes and sizes. Some lifelike. Some shaped like rabbits or toy soldiers. Some insertable. Some not. Many are designed for stimulating specific areas—the clitoris or G-spot, for example, or both at the same time. Some even feature special devices for simultaneous clitoral, G-spot, and anal stimulation. Vibrators range in price from $8 to $80.

Your main choice when selecting a vibrator is whether it should plug in or be battery operated. The best-selling model year after year at Good Vibrations in San Francisco is the Hitachi Magic Wand, a long-handled electric vibrator with a soft round head. It is also available in a rechargeable model, so you can enjoy it without getting tangled up in wires.

## CLEAN AND HEALTHY

**Using a dildo or vibrator is a good safe-sex option. Just make sure you wash it thoroughly or put a condom on it before transferring it from the anus to the vagina or mouth. Better yet, put a condom on it any time you use it. The same advice goes for using a finger or your penis in the anal area: Don't put it in other orifices without washing it thoroughly first or changing the condom. The anus hosts bacteria that can cause infections elsewhere.**

Battery-operated vibrators are less expensive and generally more portable, though they are less durable and powerful. If your partner likes a good buzz, you also can treat her to a hands-free vibrator, which fits snugly against her clitoris with a jockstrap-like harness. The newest version, the Audi-Oh, is activated by sound. You can plug it into your stereo to let her groove to the music, or you can sweet-talk her into bliss Barry White–style. Hands-free vibrators also can be worn during intercourse. That way, you can enjoy the vibrations, too.

**DILDOS.** Taking their name from the Italian *diletto,* meaning "delight," these toys are designed for insertion. They range in size from pinkie-finger small to overgrown-zucchini large. Though most are shaped like the real deal, they also come in nonanatomical shapes like a whale or dolphin. Some vibrate and have extra protrusions for clitoral and/or anal stimulation. You can buy a simple rubber dildo for about $15, but for top quality, go with a silicone model (prices average about $30 to $40). They're easier to clean, and, unlike cold rubber, silicone retains body heat and feels better during play.

**ANAL PLUGS.** These smaller members of the dildo family are expressly designed for anal stimulation, which both you and your partner can enjoy either during intercourse or solo. What makes anal plugs special is that they have a flared base to prevent them from getting caught in the rectum. Start with the smallest one you can find and work your way to a larger size over time. Insert the toy gently, using liberal amounts of lubrication to avoid tearing delicate anal and rectal tissue. Let the toy just sit there at first, responding to normal body movement. After a while, when the sensation becomes comfortable, try gently moving it in and out. Anal plugs cost about $15.

**BALLS AND BEADS.** Ben wa balls have been enjoyed in Asian countries for more than a thousand years. These golf ball–size toys are hollow and contain another ball inside, which provides a pleasant "thumping" sensation as they bump against one another inside a woman's vagina. For anal stimulation, try anal beads— marble-size silicone beads threaded together on a string and secured in place with a silicone ring. They can be inserted before intercourse or oral sex, then gently pulled out one at a time for intense stimulation during orgasm. Balls and beads range in price from $5 to $25.

**RINGS AND SLEEVES.** Though most sex toys are created for women, these you can call your own. Most notable in this category is the constriction device, or cock ring. By placing the ring at the base of your erection, you trap blood in the erectile chamber and stay hard longer. Though these toys can enhance your pleasure, don't get carried away with them. Constrictor rings cut off fresh blood flow to your penis and should never be worn longer than 20 minutes, or you risk serious tissue damage. To avoid injury, get one that is made of soft leather or latex and adjustable with Velcro, snaps, or a bolo tie.

"Sleeves" slide over the penis to provide a snug, warm, moist sensation (like the real thing) during manual stimulation. Some even vibrate. Rings and sleeves run about $5 to $20.

**LUBRICANTS.** Designed to make caressing and insertion more sensuous and slippery, lubricants can be used with sex toys or by themselves during intercourse and massage. The women we spoke to love their lubes. "*Lubricants cut down on friction and soreness after a lo-o-ong, fun time,*" explained a 25-year-old Denver graduate student. "*The commercial varieties are almost better than what nature has provided,*" confessed a 33-year-old paralegal from St. Louis. They come in a wide variety, too. You'll find body rubs in every flavor and scent. There are even special heating oils that warm up when you blow on them. At just $3 a pop, they're a cheap, easy way to spice up everyday sex.

**GAMES**. If your partner is a little shy about sexual experimentation, a sex game can be a great way to break the ice. Designed with women in mind, board and dice games are short on rules and shorter on competition, offering gentle ways to coax her into being sexually adventurous. Most board games just ask you to do little erotic things that seem silly but encourage communication, along with arousal. For example, a card may tell you, "Touch your partner somewhere you've never touched before." Or you may land on a space and be instructed to spread whipped cream on your body where you'd like your partner to lick it off.

## BACKDOOR PLAY

According to a *Redbook* study of 100,000 women, 43 percent of women have tried anal sex with their partners at least once. Not surprisingly, about half did not enjoy it. Forty percent reported finding pleasure in this still stigmatized sex act, and the remaining women gave it neither yay nor nay.

Though anal sex sounds difficult and uncomfortable, if not painful, it *does* have the potential to be quite enjoyable. That's because the lining of the anal cavity is brimming with feel-good nerve endings that add pleasure to foreplay and intercourse when stimulated. For the man, the tightness of the anus can provide a new, powerful sensation during intercourse.

Facts and stats aside, don't be surprised if your partner puts the kibosh on backdoor exploration. If you're curious, approach the subject—and the act—carefully and gently. If she doesn't react with a straight-armed forget-about-it, chances are she's game to try, if just once. One woman who told us she enjoyed anal stimulation offered this advice, "*Go slow! A glass of wine helps everyone relax. Lots of good lubricant is a must. Using a very small dildo first can help. If she says 'no more' at any time, stop immediately.*" Other tips:

**START CLEAN.** Showering or bathing together before anal sex will help you both get as clean as possible inside and out.

## SCORE A HAT TRICK

Most of us rely on the clitoris like the automatic garage door opener. It's a go-to button to gain rumbling access when we want to park our car. But there's more to the female orgasm than massage, rub, repeat. Though clitoral stimulation provides a reliable orgasm, your partner may experience intense, multiple, simultaneous orgasms if you stimulate two—or three—of her hot spots at the same time.

Next time you're manually or orally stimulating your partner's clitoris, insert a finger in her vagina and locate the rough, raised G-spot on the front of her vaginal wall. Stimulate both with about equal pressure until she comes to a shuddering "bigasm"—an orgasm that comes from both erogenous zones.

Then take it to the next level. Following the same directions as above, use your other hand to reach under her and gently stimulate her anal area with your fingertips. The resulting "trigasm" will deliver a high-voltage, full-body release. With some maneuvering, you can achieve the same result during intercourse. In the woman-on-top position, have her tilt her hips forward so that your penis hits her G-spot and her clitoris is rubbing against your shaft with every thrust. Then reach around and simultaneously stimulate her anal area with your fingertips.

**ASK FIRST.** Never just wander a finger or your penis to that general area and start poking around. That's likely to elicit a clamp-down.

**PROTECT YOURSELF.** Even if you and your partner have been together since the dinosaurs and are 100 percent disease free, you should wear a condom during anal sex to prevent getting an infection from the bacteria in the rectum. A well-lubricated condom will also be easier on her during insertion.

**LUBRICATE LIBERALLY.** The rectum is not a self-lubricating area like the vagina. It is also *much* more susceptible to painful tearing. Apply a water-based lubricant like K-Y Jelly to yourself and to her before you start. Add more as needed.

**USE SUPER SLOW-MO.** She must be completely relaxed and receptive if there is any hope for successful anal sex. That means taking your time. Start with your pinkie finger or a small dildo. Work up to just the tip of your penis. Once inside, ease in as slowly as possible or let her bear down on you. If she says enough, stop then and there. If she wants out, pull out. Once you get to the point of thrusting, do so slowly and very, very gently.

## TIE ME UP, TIE ME DOWN

Power-play sex has gotten a bad rap in popular entertainment. In Stephen King's *Gerald's Game,* a woman is left cuffed in a remote cabin after her kink-loving hubby bites it during rough sex. In *Basic Instinct,* the tables turn, and it's the men who take it to heart (literally) with an ice pick while submitting to a little tie-and-tease action. But the truth is, plenty of perfectly normal, nonhomicidal couples enjoy a little playful bondage and discipline (B&D) now and then.

*"Bondage of any kind requires a lot of trust. If that trust is there, not being able to see what's coming next can be very exciting,"* says a 44-year-old medical worker from suburban Philadelphia. *"Tell her*

*exactly what you are going to do, step by step (no pain, please, unless she's into it). The anticipation will get her so wet you can forget about lubes."* The key word here, though, is *trust*. A surprising number of women we talked to, even happily married ones who gleefully dallied with dildos and anal play, took a step back at the suggestion of being tied up. More than a few said simply, *"I'm not trusting enough."*

Because bondage and discipline treads into sensitive areas of power and control, it's not only essential that you get your partner's consent, it may be necessary for you to show your trust by giving her the ties first. She will likely be more comfortable and willing to play along when she has the pleasure of calling the initial shots.

Before you embark on any B&D adventure, agree on a code word that means "Stop now. I've had enough." Having such a signal (called a safeword in bondage lingo) leaves you free to scream and beg and bully as much as you want to as part of the fun, knowing that the one and only safeword will put an end to things if they get too rough or one of you starts feeling uncomfortable.

Some people like to throw a little sadomasochism (S&M) into the mix. Many women (and men) enjoy gentle spanking and nipple squeezing during foreplay and intercourse. But don't pull out the leather riding crop unless you've talked it over ahead of time. Any unpleasant surprises can result in a big sexual setback.

The sexually adventurous can buy elaborate handcuffs, blindfolds, and harnesses for all this naughty play. But homemade restraints (silk scarves, neckties) work just as well and don't need to be hidden from friends and family.

## FANTASY IN REALITY

You were just there to mow the lawn, maybe plant a few petunias, and there she was, the hot, horny housewife lying by the pool, wearing nothing but a silk scarf and a come-and-get-me smile. Her husband could come home at any minute, but who can resist 10 minutes of afternoon delight? After you're done, you can be a hardened criminal, and she'll be the warden. Or a pilot and a flight attendant. Therein lies the beauty of fantasy—it gives your subconscious a chance to play games limited only by your imagination.

Experts have different theories on the origin of sexual fantasy. Some say it's our brains playing out desires we've accumulated since birth. Others argue that sexual daydreams are a survival mechanism of sorts—a way of playing out situations that could be immoral, dangerous, or illegal. The one point they all agree on: We all have them, and we should simply enjoy them rather than reading too much into what it all means.

One way to enjoy this mental sexual theater is to do what we all already do—use them as fodder for masturbation. It also can be fun to bring them to life in a safe way by role playing with your partner. The biggest barrier here is embarrassment. Many women feel awkward or just plain stupid dressed up as French maids. But if you can help your partner through her inhibitions, often by taking the first step yourself, she may be willing to play along.

One cautionary note: When sharing your fantasies, use common sense. You may regard your interest in riding reverse cowgirl with the local lifeguard as an innocent diversion of the mind, but she may mistake it as an actual desire to stray. Communicate, play it smart, and keep your fantasy exploits anonymous. Or better yet, let her take center stage in your most erotic theatrics. Some popular fantasies to play out:

**FOOTBALL PLAYER AND HEAD CHEERLEADER.** Lift her skirt and go for a score.

**BUSINESS EXECUTIVE AND SEXY INTERN.** Call a private meeting and ask her to take some very personal dictation.

**TEACHER AND STUDENT.** She's Mrs. Robinson, and you're a very bad boy.

**NURSE AND PATIENT.** A kiss and caress for wherever it hurts.

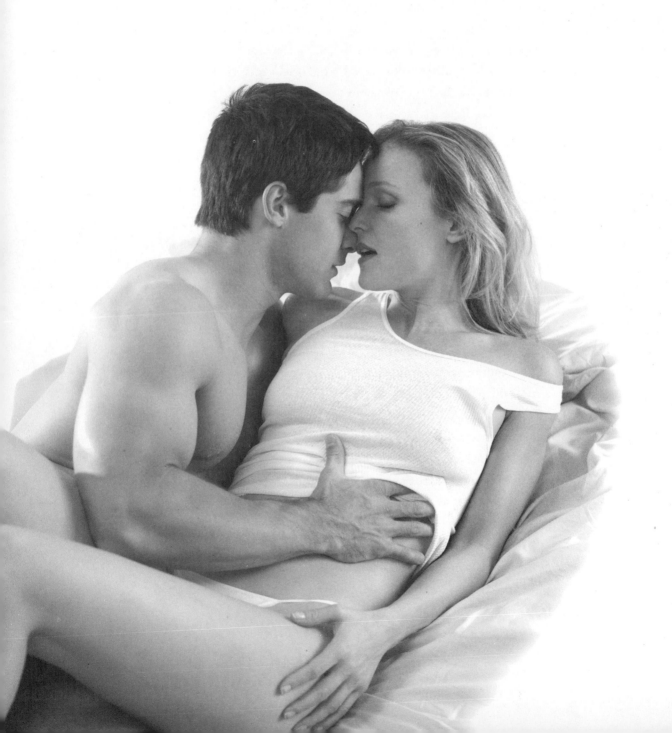

▼

**PART 2**

# MAXIMIZE PLEASURE CONTROL

# CHAPTER 3

# HARDER, LONGER

**HOW LONG DOES IT TAKE YOU TO COME DURING SEX? IF YOU'RE LIKE MOST MEN, YOU PROBABLY CLOCK IN AT AROUND 3 MINUTES.** That's fine for a quickie, but not necessarily long enough for over-the-top enjoyment—yours as well as hers. How about your erections? Are they hard enough for satisfying sex? Again, the average man has some issues in this area. Between 20 and 30 million American men can't perform the way they'd like, and we *all* have trouble from time to time.

Obviously, every man responds differently to erotic stimulation, and context always makes a difference: your mood, how much you've had to drink, the quality of your relationship with your partner, and so on. Some men ejaculate almost immediately after starting sex, and if they've had good foreplay and are in a comfortable relationship, they might be perfectly happy with their performance. Another man might last 5, 10, or 20 minutes and be disappointed that he came so quickly.

There's so much individual variation in sexual expectations and performance that it's a stretch to call anything normal. But we know in our guts that we're supposed to perform in certain ways, and we feel a sting of disappointment when we don't. Worse, the penis—and by extension, a man's perception of his sexual performance—is often the butt of lame jokes in a way that a woman's genitals or performance aren't. We might laugh when someone makes a joke about a "pencil dick" or being too "quick on the trigger," but behind the laughter, there's a lot of sexual anxiety.

Curiously, it's men themselves who create much of the stress. Women, numerous surveys show, are relatively unconcerned about the size of a man's penis, how long he lasts, or whether he's always hard and ready.

*"We have anxiety of our own about our bodies being judged and whether or not we'll be able to have an orgasm,"* says a 29-year-old marine biologist in Galveston, Texas, who responded to our survey. *"Men should relax and know that getting there is just as much fun."*

Indeed, men who learn how to relax, who accept the fact that their bodies aren't machines that can be programmed to perform on command, generally have fewer problems with erections or too-early ejaculation than those who work themselves up into sweaty knots of anxiety. In addition, every man can learn to improve just about every parameter of sexual performance, such as the frequency and duration of erections, how hard erections get, and how long he lasts during sex. An obvious point, one that we frequently overlook, is that the penis *is* a machine of sorts, just as your muscles are machines, and can be improved with specific exercises.

The vast majority of men don't need a whole lot of work to kick their sexual performance up a notch or two. We're talking a couple of minutes a day at most—and as you'll see, they'll be some of the most pleasurable minutes you've ever experienced.

## ANATOMY OF AN ERECTION

The penis carries way too much emotional baggage, especially when you consider that on the purely physical level, it's mainly a conduit for urine and semen and is made up largely of nerves, muscles, and blood.

Let's start with the issue of size. The average man has about 6 inches of *visible* penis. The other half is rooted deep inside the body, extending nearly back to the anus. The "root" of the penis, which ducks under the prostate gland, forks into two branches that attach to the pelvic bone, which holds the whole thing in place.

### INSIDE THE PENIS

The penis is more than 50 percent muscle, and a hefty percentage of that muscle is found in the tiny blood vessels that lace through it like lines on a road map. It's no accident that the penis is blood-rich terrain. When you're sexually aroused, signals from the brain (or

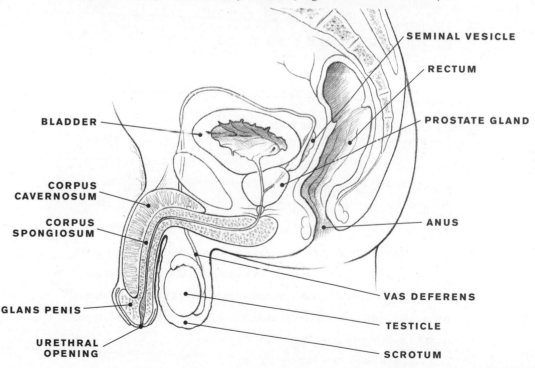

SEMINAL VESICLE

RECTUM

PROSTATE GLAND

BLADDER

CORPUS CAVERNOSUM

CORPUS SPONGIOSUM

ANUS

GLANS PENIS

VAS DEFERENS

URETHRAL OPENING

TESTICLE

SCROTUM

from the penis itself) tell blood vessels to relax. Blood flows through the tissues and gets temporarily locked in place, causing an erection.

Let's say you're spending a quiet night at home watching TV. Your thumb, apparently with a mind of its own, clicks to a cable channel featuring a little adult entertainment. The movie is hot, and your brain responds by sending stimuli down neural pathways all the way to your penis. Blood pours into the corpora cavernosa, the tubes of tissue that constitute the core of the penis. Within minutes or less, the amount of blood in the penis can increase by a factor of 10. At the same time, the expanding penile tissues squeeze against blood vessel walls and prevent blood from getting out. If you're generally healthy, you're probably pretty hard at this point—and will stay that way until the sexy nerve transmissions stop.

Nature takes erections seriously. To make sure they occur, there are two separate nerve pathways to the penis. The first comes into

## "BLUE BALLS": FACT OR FANCY?

Generations of eager men have tried to shame generations of reluctant women into having sex by playing victim politics: "Honey, we have to have sex right now to get rid of this *agonizing* pain."

There is a kernel of truth to these protestations of pain, but just barely. When a man is sexually aroused, blood flows into the penis and testicles, then just as quickly flows out when he comes. However, blood leaves the scene more slowly when he doesn't ejaculate. The pressure from accumulated blood can in fact make the testicles a little achy.

However, the discomfort rarely lasts longer than a few minutes, and it's hardly agonizing. A guy who truly feels uncomfortable can always go home and take care of things himself. In most cases, though, he doesn't need relief at all, just a little patience. Insisting makes for lousy sex—and worse relationships.

play when, say, you or your partner strokes your penis. An erection can occur pretty much automatically, whether or not you're thinking sexy thoughts. It's just a basic reflex. The second pathway travels directly from the brain and is triggered by erotic thoughts—the kind generated by the aforementioned adult movie, for example.

The best erections, those that are hardest and feel best, usually involve signals from *both* nervous pathways working in delightful harmony.

## MORE BLOOD, MORE PLEASURE

Okay, so you need blood, a lot of it, to get and maintain a good erection. A lot of men, especially those 40 and older, simply don't get enough. Psychological factors such as stress or performance anxiety can certainly cause problems, but they aren't the main culprits. Doctors estimate that about 70 percent of men who suffer frequent erection problems have an underlying vascular problem or diseases that affect nerves as well as bloodflow, such as diabetes.

No man wants to discuss sexual problems with anyone, including doctors. Do it anyway. For one thing, the vast majority of men who aren't performing the way they'd like can improve dramatically with medical treatment, counseling, or a combination of both. Why suffer in bed if you don't have to? More important, some of the same conditions that restrict bloodflow to the penis can also impede circulation to other parts of the body, such as the heart. You've got to find out what's going on, or you could find yourself with more to worry about than an erection—like a heart attack.

Since the focus of this chapter is on ways to make erections (and orgasms) better and more reliable, this isn't the place to dwell on the many causes and treatments of full-fledged erection problems. That said, almost any man will notice an improvement in sexual vigor if he does a few simple things.

**WHACK THE WINGS.** The usual nutritional advice is about as interesting as front-row seats at the World Shuffleboard Invitational. But there's a good reason that doctors almost beg guys to eat at least five daily servings of vegetables, along with plenty of fruit—and to cut back on the buffalo wings and Krispy Kremes. The more fat and cholesterol you have sloshing around in your blood, the more likely you are to wake up one day with thick, sticky deposits on the walls of your arteries. The blood vessels that you need for erections are a lot smaller than the pipes leading to the heart. Even a small amount of sludge can cause a lot of sexual embarrassment.

**GIVE UP THE SMOKES.** Not "someday"—now. Smoking vastly increases the rate of atherosclerosis, nature's equivalent of blood vessel cement. The equation, remember, boils down to this: Bad bloodflow = bad erections.

**CHECK YOUR MEDS.** Dozens of prescription drugs can take the heat out of your sexual furnace. If you're having erection problems and are taking antidepressants, tranquilizers, appetite suppressants, or ulcer drugs such as Tagamet (cimetidine), have a chat with your doc. Switching to a different drug will probably deliver the same benefits without the sexual downside.

**LOG SOME COUCH TIME.** Yes, it's uncomfortable at first to discuss intimate problems with a therapist, and yes, it can be expensive, but there's a reason that psychologists drive expensive cars. About 10 to 20 percent of erection problems are caused, at least in part, by psychological issues. Therapists who specialize in sexual problems such as

▼

**Men of the French Renaissance aristocracy thought that they could increase penis size by hanging money bags from their erections. They'd keep adding gold coins or jewels until the bag slid off. They believed that the penis had reached its optimal size when the bag stayed in place for 2 minutes.**

▲

impotence have a very high success rate at restoring normal performance.

**EXERCISE DAILY.** No kidding, it makes a difference. For one thing, regular exercise, even if it's nothing more strenuous than walking for half an hour, improves bloodflow throughout the body, including in the penis. It also stimulates a surge in endorphins, those "happy" brain chemicals that dispel stress and make you feel mentally strong and confident—the keys to good sex.

## THE ORGASMIC EDGE

An orgasm is one of those ineffable sensations that are impossible to put into words. So we won't even try; you know what it feels like. The issue for most men is how to control the timing of orgasms a little better, giving yourself and your partner a little more pleasure.

If you find that you come more quickly than you want to—keeping in mind that uncommonly steamy sex can give any man a hair trigger—you can literally train your penis to respond a little more slowly. In other words, it takes practice.

It's true. Men who deliberately take themselves through the whole sexual cycle—arousal and erection followed by a controlled orgasm—can learn to hold off to a surprising degree. You don't want to take this too far, of course. Myths to the contrary, most women don't appreciate a man who tirelessly pounds away like a piston. It makes them sore, not excited. But ejaculatory control—whether that means lasting 5 minutes or 30—is one of the best gifts you can give yourself and your lover.

You can certainly improve ejaculatory control with lovemaking, but practice during masturbation is more effective because you can concentrate entirely on your body's responses rather than being distracted by the needs of your partner. The idea is to make masturbation a long, disciplined process, one that deliberately slows the sprint to orgasm. Here's what to do.

**GIVE YOURSELF TIME.** A lot of time. If you're like most men, you probably masturbate quickly, more to get rid of sexual tension than to languorously enjoy every moment. This approach almost guarantees a quick release—and trains your body accordingly.

**TURN THE PROCESS AROUND.** The next time you're in the mood, allow at least as much time for masturbation as you would if you were having sex with your partner. Foreplay with yourself? Why not? Set the mood: Dim the lights; spin some tunes. Touch yourself lightly, even casually at first. Savor the first tinglings of excitement. Once you're hard, see how long you can stay that way without coming. Keep the hot mental images flowing through your head, but don't let them take you over the top.

**SQUEEZE TO STOP.** When you feel that you're reaching the point of no return, stop doing whatever it is you're doing and firmly squeeze the frenulum, the sensitive part of the penis just below the head. Maintain the pressure until you no longer feel that you're about to come. Then s-l-o-w-l-y resume the strokes that got you there in the first place.

**TAKE YOURSELF FORWARD AND BACK.** Keep touching yourself until you feel like you're almost ready to come, then back off by squeezing the frenulum. Repeat the process at least two or three times—more often as you gain more control. The idea isn't only to delay your orgasm at the moment but also to train your body's responses to sexual stimulation. Just as you can lift progressively heavier weights every week that you go to the gym, you can train the penis to respond more slowly and with better control.

**TAKE THE LESSONS TO REAL LIFE.** The next time you're having sex, whether that involves touch, oral contact, or intercourse, practice the same start/stop technique. When you're about to come, grip the top of your penis, squeeze until the anticipatory feelings of orgasm fade, then start again.

You'll probably need to use the squeeze technique for awhile. Eventually you'll also gain more *mental* control of impending orgasms. Your penis—and the brain signals that fire it—won't demand the same immediate release that they did before. You'll last longer just by wanting to. That's good news for you and your partner.

When things don't work out as planned, as inevitably happens, put it out of your head. Too many men get so wound up by worries about sexual performance that they simply can't perform. Take seriously this advice from a 29-year-old woman, a newspaper reporter in Miami: *"Not being able to perform has a lot more to do with what's going on in your head than in your groin. If it's not happening, don't force it, and don't get upset about it. Tell me a fantasy that will get you going, and I'll act it out. Or just relax and let me*

## SPANK YOUR CANCER RISK

Here's another argument in favor of masturbation: New research suggests that it may prevent cancer.

Australian researchers asked more than 2,500 men, ages 20 to 50, about their sexual habits. They found that those who ejaculated the most, more than five times a week, were a third less likely to get prostate cancer later in life.

Researchers speculate that ejaculation is a kind of flushing mechanism. A man's semen absorbs high concentrations of potassium, zinc, citric acid, and other substances from the blood. At the same time, it picks up potential carcinogens. A man who ejaculates frequently may be less vulnerable to cancer-causing cell changes.

The key seems to be masturbating; intercourse may not have the same effect. Ejaculation during sex with a partner does purge the prostate, but if you have multiple partners, you increase your risk of exposure to sexually transmitted diseases, which can increase prostate cancer risk by up to 40 percent.

*give you a massage. The key is relaxing and getting your mind off it. Take away the pressure and let things happen naturally."*

## A TOTAL-CONTROL WORKOUT

One simple type of exercise, traditionally recommended by doctors to women patients, can make a tremendous difference for men who ejaculate more quickly than they'd like. The exercises, known as Kegels, improve ejaculatory control and can make an erection stronger and harder.

## LIMITED INSURANCE

A condom will greatly minimize the odds that you'll catch a nasty disease—but it won't reduce the risk to zero.

Even though condom manufacturers follow stringent quality-control guidelines, you're still talking about a micro-thin sheath of rubber. Snagging a condom with a sharp fingernail can breach the delicate barrier. So can putting on a condom too roughly. Rubber breaks down over time, so condoms that were perfectly good when you bought them might be less than reliable a few years later.

Even if you use a condom with all its integrity intact, there's always the chance that it will work its way off during sex. There is also the unpleasant possibility of an unforeseen explosion—not to mention infection from diseases that don't depend strictly on genital-to-genital contact, such as herpes or venereal warts.

To play it safe, you're better off using latex condoms than "skins." Synthetic materials have smaller pores, which reduce the risk that an elusive microbe will slip through. Pay attention to what you're doing when putting on a condom. Work gently, and definitely remove it as soon as you're done having sex. A condom that fits firmly on an erection is like a loose pair of jeans once you get soft.

First developed by Los Angeles gynecologist Arnold Kegel, MD, the exercise is designed to strengthen the pubococcygeus (PC) muscle in the pelvis. The PC wraps around the base of the penis and the anus and reflexively contracts during orgasm. Making the muscle stronger makes it easier to delay orgasms and makes them stronger and more intense.

The exercise itself couldn't be simpler. All you have to do is contract the PC muscle—the same one that you'd use to stop the flow of urine in midstream. Hold the contraction for 2 or 3 seconds, inhaling as you squeeze. Relax for a moment, then squeeze again. Do the exercise in sets of 10 at first, then increase the number to 20 or 30 squeezes. Repeat the sequence several times a day.

▼

**"The good thing about masturbation is that you don't have to dress up for it."**

**—TRUMAN CAPOTE,** *American writer*

▲

Once you've developed strength in the PC, you'll find that it's easy to stop an orgasm just by contracting it. It's easier and more convenient than the "squeeze" technique for stopping an orgasm during masturbation. Another key difference is that Kegels not only delay orgasm but actually build muscle at the same time—an important point because about 85 percent of men can't have intercourse for longer than 3 minutes, largely due to an underdeveloped PC.

To start a Kegels plan, here's what doctors advise.

**GET INTO TRAINING.** When you first start doing Kegels, you'll probably find that you're able to delay orgasm by only a slight margin, if that. That's okay. Like any workout, Kegels require persistent practice. If nothing else, you get in the habit of locating and contracting the muscles at the key time. Most men need to practice Kegels for at least 3 to 4 weeks before they notice significant changes in their ability to hold back.

**DO THEM ALL DAY.** Don't wait until you're having sex to start building the PC muscle. To build maximum strength, you need to do sets of Kegels at least three times a day, working up to about 300 forceful squeezes daily. Doing this for a month or two will greatly strengthen the PC. At this point, you'll notice improvements in your staying power as well as in the pleasurable force of your orgasms.

**DO THEM ANYWHERE.** You don't have to change into workout clothes to do Kegel exercises. You can do them anywhere: while sitting on the sofa watching TV, standing in a checkout line, or leaning over the sink and scrubbing 3-day-old pasta sauce out of your favorite pot.

**SHAKE THINGS UP.** Bored with simple Kegels? Push yourself a little harder with these variations:

▶ Slow Kegels. Tighten the PC and hold for a slow count of three. Relax, then repeat 10 or more times.

▶ Quick Kegels. Tighten and relax the PC as many times as you can in 10 seconds.

▶ Big-move Kegels. Tighten your entire abdomen and the pelvic floor muscle, then force the pressure outward by bearing down.

▶ Fluttering Kegels. Quickly tighten and relax the PC using a fluttering movement for 10 seconds. Relax for 10 seconds, then repeat.

**TAKE THE TOWEL TEST.** A pleasurable way to test the strength of the PC is to see how successful you are at pulling back from the brink of orgasm. Here's another self-test: The next time you have an erection, hang a small bath towel on your penis and try to move it up and down. You won't have any trouble if the PC is strong. You can also use this exercise to make the muscle even stronger. Can you raise and lower the towel 100 times? The same movement inside your partner will give her an added bit of pleasure.

**ALLOW SOME DOWNTIME.** Working the PC with Kegels, like any other form of exercise, can leave you a little sore at first. Some discomfort is normal, but why live with it? Do Kegels for a few days, then take a day off to allow the muscle to flush out accumulations of pain-causing lactic acid. Then start the program again.

## POWER TO THE PELVIS

You can't build a house with a hammer alone, and you can't have great sex just because you have a strong erection. You also have to have strong supporting muscles, especially those that attach to the pelvic girdle, the bony arch that supports your legs.

Sex, as Elvis showed shocked parents a generation ago, is all in the pelvis. Your partner will notice the difference when you're strong and limber enough to swivel and twist. A strong pelvis means that you can hold sexual positions, especially those that involve sitting, for a longer time, without straining your back or depending on your arms for support.

As with any stretching program, you can do the following pelvic workouts pretty much anywhere, even on your office floor if you can get away with it. Better yet, do them with your partner. Women benefit from a stronger pelvis just as much as men do, and doing the stretches together will add an erotically charged dimension to your relationship.

STRETCHES: POWER TO THE PELVIS

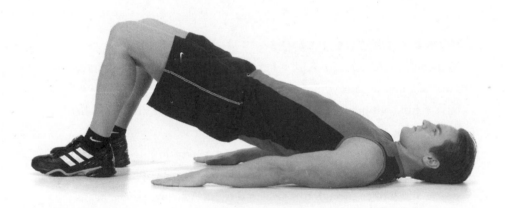

## PELVIC LIFT

**START:** Lie on your back with your knees bent and slightly apart. Your feet should be flat on the floor and your arms at your sides.

**FINISH:** Inhale, firmly clench your abs and butt, and lift your pelvis until your spine is straight but not arched. Breathe out, hold for at least 10 seconds, then relax and repeat.

## STRETCHES: POWER TO THE PELVIS

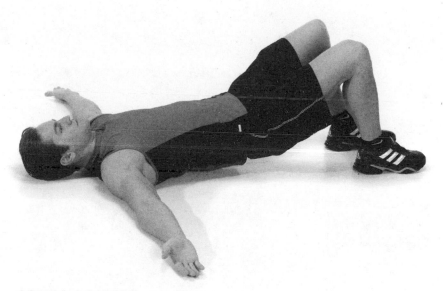

## PELVIC BOUNCE

**START:** Lie on your back with your knees bent and slightly apart. Extend your arms to the sides with the palms facing up.

**FINISH:** Inhale, lifting your pelvis just slightly off the floor. Hold for a few seconds, then lower yourself so that your lower back lightly touches the floor. Relax, then repeat. Exhale and let down so your lower back bounces gently against the floor.

## STRETCHES: POWER TO THE PELVIS

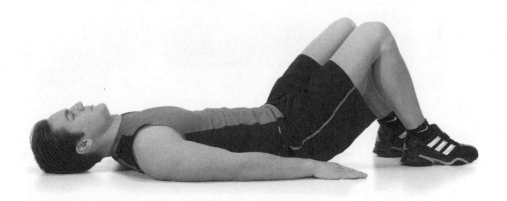

### PELVIC TILT

**START:** Lie on your back with your knees bent. Your feet should be flat on the floor and your arms at your sides.

**FINISH:** Clench your abs and butt tightly while firmly pressing your lower back against the floor. Hold for 3 to 5 seconds, then relax and repeat.

## STRETCHES: POWER TO THE PELVIS

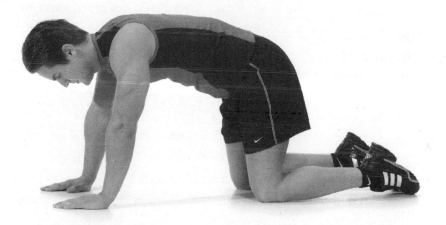

## HORSE STANCE

**START:** Get on your hands and knees, with your elbows locked and your hands under your shoulder blades. Flatten your lower back and drop your shoulder blades.

**FINISH:** Pull your navel toward your spine and hold for about 90 seconds, then relax.

### FINDING THE MULTIPLE O

Many women enjoy the unique pleasure of having multiple orgasms. This experience, alas, is denied to most men. When a man ejaculates, he naturally slips into a refractory period—the resting stage in which the body slowly prepares for more action. He's down for the count, in other words.

But some men do have multiple orgasms. The secret to their enjoyment lies in the fact that orgasm and ejaculation are two distinct events. Within limits, many men can teach themselves to experience orgasms without the out-rush of semen. Retaining semen during orgasm is the secret to coming again—and with luck, again and again. Some men report having three or four orgasms in succession, without interruption or loss of sexual arousal.

▼

**Sex researcher Dr. Alfred Kinsey estimated that the average man thinks about sex roughly every 5 minutes.**

▲

The ability to come repeatedly isn't as elusive as you might think. Then again, not every man can do it. It's really determined by the roll of your individual physiological dice. But anything that feels so good is certainly worth a try. Here's what you need to do.

**GET COMFORTABLE.** *Real* comfortable. A study by Marian E. Dunn, PhD, of the State University of New York Health Science Center in Brooklyn, found that most multi-orgasmic men had sex with women they knew well and were comfortable with. They also had their best moments when the atmosphere and circumstances surrounding sex were relaxed and stress-free. At the same time, it's helpful to periodically stimulate the entire penis, along with the scrotum and the perineum (the area between the anus and penis), to heighten sexual arousal.

**STRENGTHEN THE PCS.** They have to be strong to hold back the rush of semen when you come. Doing frequent Kegels throughout the day is essential if you hope to ride the multi-train.

**SQUEEZE LIKE HELL WHEN THE MOMENT COMES.** Either clench the PC when you feel an orgasm is imminent or use your hand to squeeze the top of your penis. You have to stop yourself from ejaculating, however tempting it might be to let go.

**FOCUS ON THE SENSATIONS.** Once you're able to back off when you're ready to come, pay special attention to what you're feeling. You may notice what experts call contractile phase orgasms, sensations that are very similar to, if more subtle than, regular orgasms. With practice, these "mini-orgasms" may be just as powerful as your former orgasms, with the special bonus of lasting longer.

# CHAPTER 4

# MASTERING TOTAL CONTROL

**WE RECENTLY HEARD FROM A 47-YEAR-OLD FIREFIGHTER IN OMAHA.** He might be bragging a bit, but his note illustrates better than we ever could the connection between physical fitness and great sex: *"For the average couple, unless they're in great shape, I would think they would have a hard time achieving the duration, intensity, and number and type of positions that my girlfriend and I experience."*

There's no deep mystery about why spending a few hours a week in the gym enhances libido as well as performance. Working out lowers levels of stress hormones. It can transform your heart into a pounding drum and your arteries into forceful conduits. It increases energy, improves sleep, and boosts levels of testosterone. You've heard all of this before, but it's definitely worth repeating because we can all use a little convincing to get off the couch and do—*anything*.

Strength training and cardiovascular conditioning are just one part of fitness. You also need a high degree of *sexual* fitness if you hope to have the kinds of intimate encounters that can fill your head with fantasies. This is the one area where nearly all men need some help. Even if you're physically capable of having the kind of sex you want—you get easy erections, don't tire easily, and so on—you might not have the specific skill sets to make sex last as long as you'd like or have the kind of mind-blowing orgasms that you dream about.

In the following pages, we'll explain, step by step, how to dramatically increase sexual endurance. How to come exactly when you want and not before. How to increase orgasmic intensity so that it rivals the multiple orgasms some women take for granted. These aren't pie-in-the-sky fantasies. Scientists who study sex have developed very

## BITS AND PIECES

No matter how many times you've been around the block, there's always something new, or at least unfamiliar, in the world of sex. We asked some of the country's top researchers to share some of the little-known sexual facts that they felt every man should know. Here are their top picks.

▶ Only about a third of women come during straight intercourse. So quit feeling guilty—and put your fingers, mouth, or vibrator to work.

▶ Few women appreciate overly long sexual sessions. Making love for more than 30 minutes often causes more soreness than excitement.

▶ The average man loses and regains his erection up to four times during intercourse.

▶ The average woman is stimulated by the periodic softening of a man's penis in her vagina.

▶ Most women want a man to stay inside them as long as possible after intercourse.

▶ Men (and women) almost *have* to fall asleep after sex because the adrenal glands release a burst of epinephrine after orgasm. Epinephrine causes a temporary increase in pulse, blood pressure, and blood circulation to the muscles, which is followed by profound relaxation.

specific techniques for breathing, ejaculatory response, and muscular control. Some of these exercises are derived from clinical studies of men's sexual responses. Others are refinements of ancient sexual practices. Used together, they can take you to places you probably can't imagine now—places to which, when you look back 10 years from now, will make you wonder how you managed to be satisfied before.

## ORGASM ON DEMAND

Have you ever wondered what makes you hard? Not what actually triggers the process—that could be anything from the sight of a tight miniskirt to the sensations of jeans against skin—but how your body translates the initial "I want some of that" fantasies into mechanical action? Although it varies from one person to another, these are the four phases of male sexual response.

▶ 1. Excitement: When you first get turned on, electrical signals travel from the brain down the spinal cord and into your genitals. Blood vessels relax, and blood pours into the spongy tissue in the penis. (Two chambers of tissue, the corpora cavernosa, wrap around the top and sides of your penis; a third chamber, the corpus spongiosum, wraps around the urethra and forms the head at the top of the penis.)

▶ 2. Plateau: Once enough blood is assembled—and for men over about age 40, this generally requires direct physical stimulation in addition to erotic thoughts—nerves in the genitals release a substance that essentially shuts the gates. Rather than flowing in and out as usual, blood stays in the spongy caverns. That's what makes you hard and keeps you hard until you ejaculate.

When you're approaching the point of no return, the prostate gland, the small band that circles the urethra at the base of the bladder, tightens, then releases fluid into the urethra. At the same time, the scrotum tightens, and the testicles jam up against the body. This is the moment when you're ready to go; it's like the split second after your finger pulls the trigger on a gun and sends a bullet toward the light of day. Nothing short of instantaneous death (and maybe not even that) will stop you from coming.

▶ 3. Orgasm: The pelvic muscles tighten and force semen out of the penis. All of that accumulated blood starts to ebb. Your heart pounds, and your breathing gets heavier and faster. Blood rushes to the skin and makes you feel hot and sweaty. All the while, you're out of your head with bliss because the orgasm, for those few precious seconds, has transported you to another realm.

▶ 4. Resolution: The body returns to its prearoused state. Men generally experience a "refractory period" at the beginning of resolution, during which achieving another erection is all but impossible.

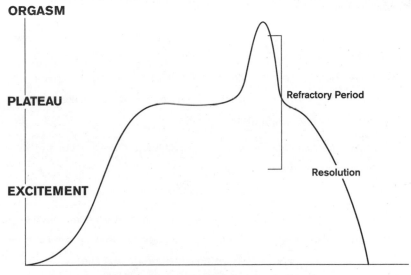

**Male Sexual Response Cycle**

The mechanics of orgasm are pretty straightforward, but the ability to control it is not. On the male anxiety meter, the idea of coming too quickly can blast you into the red zone, just behind the idea of not getting an erection. It's not a misplaced fear. Premature ejacula-

## 5 ANCIENT PLEASURE SECRETS

By taking the pressure off performance and enhancing sexual intimacy, ancient Tantric sex rituals have a great deal to offer couples today. These five are based on the 2,000-year-old body of erotic wisdom.

**Ritual.** Create a personal ritual to both celebrate and give special meaning to the sexual exchange. This might include candles, colored lights, flowers, perfumes, or a special room or bed. Also, consider expressions of affection like sensual massage or reciting poetry, or even reading erotica to each other.

**Synchronized breathing.** While touching your partner in some way, bring your breathing into sync with hers in order to create a feeling of relaxation and togetherness. Don't try too hard; instead use a "soft-focus" approach whereby you simply allow your breathing patterns to come together naturally.

**Sustained eye contact.** Though it may feel awkward at first, sustained, steady eye contact has tremendous potential for enhancing your sexual experience. Start out by doing it for a minute or two at a time, then continue as you get more comfortable with it.

**Motionless intercourse.** After you've entered her and are at a point of peak sexual arousal, become completely still. Start by doing this for a couple of minutes, then continue for longer periods.

**Refrain from orgasm.** To take the focus off performance completely, try lovemaking without orgasm. Tantric tradition suggests that avoiding or refraining from sexual release intensifies sexual/spiritual energy.

tion is among the most common problems sex therapists treat. Some men come almost immediately after entering their partners, and this can cause real problems—not only for a man's self-confidence but for his relationships as well.

Most men, though, last long enough for satisfying sex. Do they last long enough for great sex? Not often enough. The ability to *decide* when to come gives you a tremendous amount of freedom. There will be times when you and your partner, overcome by the heat of the moment, want nothing more than to explode into oblivion, the quicker the better. There will be many other times when you want to prolong the sensations, to explore a variety of positions, and to keep going and going.

Not a problem. The ability to last has very little to do with willpower and almost everything to do with technique and habit. Forget for the moment that longer sex may be its own reward. Men who train themselves to linger on the path to orgasm, who push themselves to the brink and then pull back repeatedly, generally experience greatly intensified pleasure. From a woman's point of view, your ability to last is a great bonus because it can allow her to come first while still feeling your erection inside her.

## THE TANTRIC EDGE

Unless you've taken the time to really read up on the subject, most of what you've heard about Tantric sex probably should be filed under misinformation. In essence, it's a philosophy, science, and art that promotes the creative use of sexual energy. In India, the practice of Tantric sex was first codified in the love manual *Kama Sutra* and later developed into a series of ritualized sexual positions (tantras).

In a nutshell, Tantric philosophy teaches that lovemaking, when entered into with full awareness, opens a gateway to both sexual and spiritual bliss. It treats sexual energy as something to be prolonged and savored, rather than as a performance and race to orgasm. As you might expect, the ability to control ejaculation plays a key role in Tantric sex. Men who practice it say they routinely experience multiple orgasms. Orgasm can easily be delayed half an hour or more. In the Tantric view, this languorous approach to lovemaking not only enhances pleasure but also channels sexual energy into other pursuits in life, giving more energy and self-awareness.

▼

**Until the U.S. Supreme Court struck down the nation's sodomy laws in 2003, the United States had more statutes governing sexual behavior than all the European nations combined.**

▲

You could easily spend months learning the intricacies of Tantric sex. For our purposes, the bottom line is that you can incorporate some of the approaches into your daily life to enhance all of your sexual experiences. Here are the most important steps.

**EXPAND YOUR EROTIC SENSES.** Forget the bedroom for a moment. You can't be fully sensual in bed unless you also appreciate all of life's sensuous pleasures: the silky texture of a rich, creamy soup; the brush of the wind across your face; the striking colors of autumn leaves. A man who's in touch with all of his senses, and who takes time to savor them, is a man who also knows how to appreciate the sensations of his body and those of his partner. Sex doesn't begin and end with the penis. At its best, it's an all-day affair, a kind of ongoing mental foreplay that keeps you buzzing.

**MASTURBATE OFTEN—AND TAKE YOUR TIME.** Forget the businesslike speed and force you're probably accustomed to. Men tend to masturbate to "take the edge off," which basically means going hard at it until they come. This approach certainly works if your goal is to have an orgasm in the shortest possible time, but it leaves a lot to be desired if you hope to expand your self-awareness and potential for pleasure.

The next time you masturbate, slow w-a-y down. Light a few candles. Oil up your arms and chest, enjoying the slick sensations as you rub and massage. When you move your hands to your penis, go slowly. This isn't a race. Pay attention to your emotional as well as physical feelings. More important, notice how good you feel even when you're not even close to coming. Forget the destination. Forget old habits. Good sex means throwing predictability out the window. Subtle sensations are often the most powerful, especially when you give yourself time to really explore them.

**BREATHE FOR ENDURANCE.** Most of us breathe the same way we eat: automatically, without much thought. But in Tantric sex, conscious breathing can become part of the sensual experience because it makes you intimately aware of your body. The next time you're making love, make an effort to breathe much more slowly and deeply than usual. Pay attention to each breath as it goes in and out. Apart from heightening your physical sensations, deep breathing is among the best ways to dispel the buildup of tension that can rush you too quickly to ejaculation.

**MAKE SLOW LOVE.** The best sex is meditative and very intimate. The goal isn't to maximize sensations in your penis and come quickly. Quite the opposite. You and your partner should be as relaxed as possible. Even if you're inside your partner, move as slowly as you know how. As your erotic energy builds, take a break for awhile. Give your partner a sensual massage and encourage her to caress you before starting intercourse again. Get used to savoring all of the experience, not just the climactic end.

**CLIMB THE FOUR STEPS.** The goal of Tantric sex is for lovemaking to last as long as possible by building up and backing off repeatedly.

Tantric devotees refer to the "four levels of ascent": As you make love, feel your sexual energy rising, starting with your navel and traveling upward to your heart, throat, and head. When you feel that the energy is entering the highest parts of your brain, that's the time to really let go. Men who practice this technique sometimes experience a "white light" orgasm. They feel the full, explosive rush, but don't ejaculate. With practice, you can learn to have several of these orgasms before you finally ejaculate.

## HOW MUCH VARIETY DO YOU REALLY NEED?

There are nearly as many sexual positions as there are creative couples who like to say, "Let's try this!" If you spend any time perusing the Web or erotic classics such as the *Kama Sutra,* you might get the impression that your sex life is, well, vanilla if you don't spend your Saturday nights swinging from the swag lamp.

For some people—usually the same ones who never order the same dish twice at their favorite restaurant—variety really is the spice of life. Many others, though, will regularly return to a favorite restaurant because they can get the same delicious meal they had before. They're certainly game to try something new, but for the most part, they stick to the tried and true.

So too with sex. The majority of couples stick with the same few positions that have served them well in the past and that they continue to enjoy. There's nothing boring about that.

For those adventurous souls who spend their lives seeking out the more arcane pleasures, who enjoy things most when they're obscure as well as difficult, a quick word of caution: Some of the couplings you see on porn sites are challenging, to say the least. Be careful about exploring the outer limits of sexual acrobatics unless you're also willing to devote the time to staying impressively toned and limber.

## KNOW YOUR BODY

We've talked at some length about Tantric sex because too many of us get locked into our habitual sexual responses and forget that we have the power to make them whatever we want them to be. The sexual wisdom of the East is one approach for taking control, but it's just one of many. Scientists have studied male sexual techniques and training exercises for decades. We're not talking about fuzzy concepts that are useful only if you spend your days meditating. They're very practical steps men can take to delay ejaculation and generally enjoy sex more fully.

The main reason that so many men come before they're ready is that they've never taken the time to know their bodies—to recognize the signs that say, "Whoa, it's gonna be over if I keep going." We all know what it feels like to come, but what about 30 seconds before you come? Or 2 minutes? Or 10? Having an orgasm isn't like falling off a building, even if it feels that way. A lot goes on before you get there. Once you recognize the earliest signs that the end is near and learn a few techniques for pulling back, you'll discover endurance you never knew you had. Which means more time to revel in all of the emotional and physical feelings.

The clinical term *ejaculatory inevitability* describes the point at which you're going to come, no matter what. It's during the time just before this point that you still have room to negotiate. For example, you'll probably notice these signs.

▶ Increased heart and respiratory rates. Apart from the loud breathing and pounding heart that accompany orgasms, you'll notice very gradual increases in both as your arousal rises. Unless you start out in an over-the-top state of heat, your breathing and heart rate will be close to normal when you first start making love. As the sensations get more and more pleasurable, your cardiovascular system significantly picks up the pace. This is the time to start slowing down.

▶ Contraction of the urethra. This one's pretty subtle, but you won't have any trouble feeling it when you pay attention. As you approach ejaculatory inevitability, the urethra—the tube that carries semen out of the penis—will go into pleasurable spasms. Once this happens, you don't have a lot of time. Basically, you'll have to stop whatever you're doing *immediately* if you hope to prolong the act.

▶ Increased penis size. Yep, you get bigger and usually harder as you approach orgasm. Again, you don't have a lot of time to back off once this happens—probably not much more than a few seconds if you don't slow down.

Apart from noting the sensations that accompany the climb to orgasm, it's worth keeping track of what you were doing that got you there. You probably have a good idea of the positions or movements that take you over the brink. Obviously, hard and fast sex—deep penetration and a lot of friction—will get you there fastest. The man-on-top position, because it provides the most stimulation, can trigger an early bailout for most men. The only way to truly control and expand your endurance is to get a good handle on what sets you off—and switch gears when the time is right.

## THE POWER OF BREATH

We've already touched on the concept of breathing as an important tool when you're trying to increase endurance. It's worth exploring in more detail because breathing properly—yes, there is a *right* way to do it—is among the best ways to slow your body's rush to the finish line.

Most of us use less than one-third of our lung capacity when we breathe. This means that your body, including the penis, spends most of its life on reduced oxygen rations. Since men tend to breathe quickly and shallowly during sex, especially when they get close to orgasm, the penis is starved of air right when it needs it most. This isn't a minor point. Your cells demand oxygen. Reduce the supply, and all of the cellular processes, including those that govern the expansion of arteries and permit the circulation that makes you hard, take a sudden dive in efficiency.

The mere fact that you breathe in and out doesn't count for much. You can vastly improve your air supply—and your ability to come when you want and not before—with a few quick steps.

**BREATHE YOURSELF HARD.** Before you have sex—or during, if your partner sits on top and straddles your penis—lie on your back and breathe slowly through your nose. At the same time, put your hand on your pelvis and feel it slowly rise and fall. This simple move increases arousal levels while bringing more blood to the penis.

**TIME YOUR THRUSTS.** If you spend any time at the gym, you already know that you gain power and improve oxygen intake when you exhale during the exertion phase and inhale when you relax. The same with sex. Get in the habit of thrusting inward when you exhale and breathing deeply when you pull back. You'll vastly increase your oxygen flow while at the same time gaining a significant jump in energy. As a bonus, this type of synchronized breathing dispels muscular tension and can help you hold off before coming.

**VISUALIZE AIR.** Studies have shown that you can use a technique called visualization—in which you form vivid mental images in your mind—to enhance the circulation of oxygen-rich blood to your penis as well as to muscles in your arms and legs. The same technique can also enhance the intensity of orgasms. Once a day, take about 10 minutes to do the following exercise.

▶ Lie on your back with your knees bent and your feet flat on the bed.

▶ Breathe slowly and deeply for a few seconds, then start to visualize the air entering your bloodstream and flowing into your penis. Imagine that you can feel an increase in vigor and strength.

That's all there is to it. Studies have consistently shown that athletes who practice mental imagery have better concentration as well as performance. Visualization has also been shown to significantly lower stress hormones and improve blood pressure—and good blood circulation, as you know, is essential for good sex. Not bad for a 10-minute "workout" that's all in your mind.

Incidentally, you don't have to wait until you're in bed or lying on the couch to practice deep breathing or visualization. You certainly shouldn't wait until you're already in bed with your partner. You can easily incorporate both practices into your daily life whenever you have a few seconds of downtime—while you're waiting for a light to change, in the interminable line at the bank, and so on.

## COME SLOWER, COME MORE

We talked a bit about techniques for achieving better ejaculatory control in chapter 5. They're *not* just for men who suffer from premature ejaculation. Even if your endurance is good—if, say, you can easily last 15 minutes during intercourse—you can use the same strategies to prolong lovemaking even more.

The cornerstone of any program to delay ejaculation is to repeatedly push your body to the brink and then pull back, repeating the process as often as you're able (or want to). If you do this regularly, you'll notice a dramatic improvement in your ability to "hold," possibly in as little as a few weeks. You'll probably start having orgasms that are almost mind blowing in their intensity. More than a few men who try these techniques start having multiple orgasms as well.

Here are the best techniques for ejaculatory control. Don't stick to just one; combine them for better—and faster—results.

**STEP 1: STOP AND SQUEEZE.** This is the easiest technique to delay ejaculation, although it may feel a bit unnatural at first. When you're masturbating or having sex, and you feel yourself reaching the point of orgasm, immediately stop what you're doing and firmly squeeze your penis just below the head. Continue the pressure for 15 to 30 seconds or until the urge to come subsides. Take a few deep breaths, then start again with whatever you were doing before.

▼

**The average male produces a teaspoonful of ejaculate when he comes. The protein-rich dollop contains only 5 to 25 calories.**

▲

Keep doing this—squeezing when necessary, breathing a few times, then resuming—until you're finally ready to come. Men who practice this technique regularly can often mentally pull themselves back from the brink without having to squeeze the penis each time. Of course, this works only if you stop and squeeze before you're slipping over the edge into orgasm.

**STEP 2: STOP AND GO.** When you're making love and feel that you're about ready to come, push your penis into your partner as far as you can, then stop—really stop. Press hard so that your pubic bone presses against hers. Hold this position until the urge to come passes. Resume thrusting until, once again, you reach your peak, then back off again.

**STEP 3: TENSE AND TEASE.** This is a slightly advanced technique for delaying orgasm because it requires quite a bit of muscular strength and control. Shortly before you feel yourself coming, tense the muscles hard at the base of your penis. They're the same muscles that you'd use to stop the flow of urine. Maintain the pressure until the urge passes.

This step is the hardest for men to master because they might not have well-developed pubococcygeus (PC) muscles, which stop urine as well as the flow of semen through the penis. You can bet that you'll fail the first couple of times you try it. You can accelerate your learning curve by doing Kegel exercises most days of the week. Kegels (you'll find a complete workout program starting on page 76) greatly strengthen the PC and are an essential tool in gaining better ejaculatory control.

They actually do more than that. Men who strengthen their PC muscles with Kegels and get in the habit of tensing and teasing sometimes find that they're able to experience multiple orgasms. Clamping down the PC just prior to or even during orgasms can minimize or stop ejaculation. You'll still experience the pleasurable sensations of orgasm, but without the usual rush of semen. When you take ejaculation out of the picture, you may find that you're able to experience two or even three of these "mini-orgasms" in rapid succession.

**STEP 4: PULL OUT AND STOP.** Another method for learning ejaculatory control is called the locking method, and it's based not on Tantric philosophy but on another Eastern tradition, Taoism. Here's how it works. When you feel that you're becoming too excited, simply withdraw your penis from your partner's vagina or pull back so that only the head of your penis remains inside her, then stay motionless for 10 to 30 seconds. You'll begin to lose your erection, but if you wait until the urge to ejaculate begins to subside before entering her again, you'll also begin to learn ejaculatory control. You can do this as often as you like, until you begin needing to withdraw less and less often.

Taoist masters also advised novices to practice "a thousand loving thrusts" in a variety of styles. For instance, thrust in a pattern of three slow and shallow, then one fast and deep. If you start getting too excited, just withdraw and wait for it to pass, then resume thrusting. Once you've mastered this, move on to five shallow and one deep, then nine shallow, one deep.

A final word about delaying orgasm and heightening your sense of control: Don't underestimate the power of communication. Definitely talk to your partner about what you hope to accomplish. Don't worry, she'll be all for it. And you'll need her help when you're trying to hold back a little longer. If she's doing something that's too stimulating, ask her to back off a bit. When you're ready to resume again, let her know. Working together, you'll find a comfortable sexual pattern that gives all the pleasure that you're accustomed to—and more, because you'll have the ability to enjoy it longer.

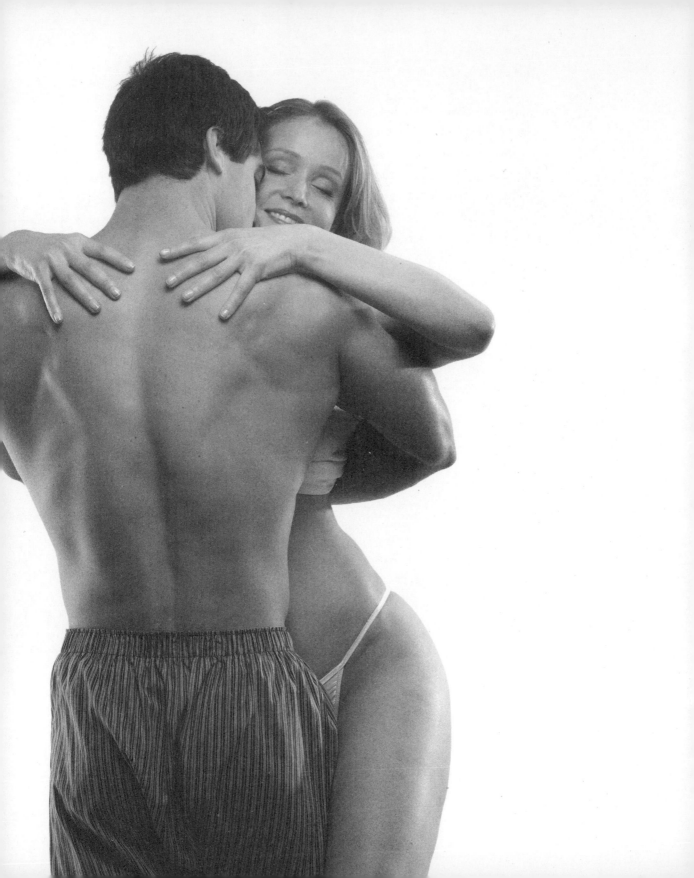

▼

**PART 3**

SEXUAL FITNESS

# CHAPTER 5

# BEND THIS WAY:
# THE ROLE OF FLEXIBILITY

**FLEXIBILITY IS ARGUABLY THE MOST IMPORTANT COMPONENT OF SEXUAL FITNESS, AND IT SEEMS TO BE THE EASIEST ONE TO IGNORE.** Let's face it, there's a deep, gut-level satisfaction in bench pressing your own weight and building a sexy chest that women love, or running every weekend to strengthen your thighs, or finding in yourself the determination to compete in a 10-K race without clutching your chest and keeling over halfway to the finish line. But stretching? B-o-r-i-n-g.

True, stretching lacks the drama and visceral thrill of competitive exercise, which is why you don't see a lot of it on ESPN. Here's something to think about, though. The benefits of flexibility go way beyond strength and endurance. To put it simply, being limber means more and better sex. You're more likely to play with new positions when your muscles move fluidly. You'll increase your partner's pleasure as well as your own when you're comfortable bending, twisting, tilting, and turning.

In less ecstatic terms, you're also less likely to get hurt when you're somewhat more limber than a saltine. Have you ever been tempted to manipulate your partner into the Hastika (elephant) pose from the *Kama Sutra* or simply to pull off a quickie in the front seat of a Neon? You'd better be flexible, or your only post-coital action will be in traction.

A letter from a *Men's Health* magazine reader amply (and painfully) illustrates this point: *"I've been trying to demonstrate to my significant other how much I appreciate her by going above and beyond in our lovemaking, but I've created a problem for myself. My desire outstrips my ability, and I end up with pains and cramps."*

Mmm, doesn't *that* sound like fun.

## FLEXIBILITY GOES FIRST

If you're like most men, you've probably noticed that your body doesn't always respond the way you want it to or the way it used to. Forget about the obvious things for a moment, such as the sad fact that your erections aren't as hard as you remember or occur more slowly and less often. On the downhill slope, flexibility is right at the top—and it keeps sliding as the decades pass.

Exercise physiologists have long noted that flexibility peaks when you're somewhere between 10 and 15 years old. In fact, you start to lose flexibility a good 15 years before the usual age-related physical declines, such as drops in muscle mass and metabolism. If you're over 35, you've probably already found yourself saying things like, "Man, I'm stiff in the morning" or "Honey, would you help me pick up my socks?"

Don't make the mistake of confusing age-related stiffness with an inevitable law of nature. Flexibility, like any other physical skill, can always be improved. Put another way, a loss of flexibility is mainly a function of how you move—or, to be honest, how you *don't* move.

Stiffness doesn't just happen. It's a consequence of not regularly pushing your muscles through their full range of motion. When you don't flex regularly, in bed or anywhere else, your muscle fibers shorten, get tighter, and snap like angry dogs when you ask them to move.

*"Simply being able to roll around while 'coupled' would be easier if we were both more flexible,"* says a 47-year-old firefighter. *"Some positions are difficult to maintain because of the awkward feelings that a lack of flexibility causes."*

It's normal, if not exactly smart, for men to focus on strength at the expense of flexibility. But you have to realize that the sexual advantages of strength, such as the ability to balance your partner on your thighs, are offset when movement is restricted by tight, stiff muscles. Sex relies much more on fluid motion than it does on brute strength. Stretching lubricates joints and makes tendons and ligaments more supple. In other words, it prepares you for the sensuous movements of sex.

▼

**Eighty-five percent of all men ejaculate in 3 minutes or less.**

▲

Here are other reasons to flex for sex.

▶ It takes only a few minutes a day, and you don't have to suit up to do it. You can even stretch with your partner before you get out of bed. Focus on shared, sensuous moments that take out the morning kinks—and that naturally transform themselves into foreplay.

▶ Stretching improves muscle growth and recovery from exercise (yes, even from sex), while at the same time enhancing sexual expression. Your muscles will work with you instead of against you.

▶ You'll feel increased sensitivity in all parts of your body when you're limber. And we do mean in *all* parts.

▶ A flexible man is a sexually creative man. You'll be more in tune with your body, more aware of what feels good—and what makes your partner feel good. Better still, you'll have the physical ability to act on your desires.

## YES, SIZE MATTERS

Of course it does. Anyone who says that size doesn't matter is either lying or has been unduly influenced by the thought police. Let's face it, a man doesn't want to be so small that he gets, well, lost during sex. Nor does he want to be so large that he threatens injury.

Between these two extremes, it all comes down to a woman's preference. The average erect penis is 6.16 inches—perfectly adequate for the vast majority of women. There will always be exceptions, of course. Vaginas, like penises, come in different shapes and sizes, and they expand and contract to different degrees. Some women like a large penis because it offers a tighter fit. Others prefer a little more room to move.

Obviously, all is relative in this domain. A man who's too large for one woman will be perfectly sized for another. One who gets lost in one woman will be custom-fit for someone else. The bottom line: Average is about right. Besides, survey after survey reports that women are far more concerned with a man's technique and enthusiasm than with penis size.

One last point: Men often worry about the length of their penises, but it's the girth that makes a bigger difference. The lower third of a woman's vagina possesses the highest concentration of nerve endings. The wider the man, the more he'll fill this area.

Men determined to "go wide" can easily achieve this by wearing a penis ring, available in any adult "toy" store, during sex. It's like tying a string around your finger. It traps more blood inside the penis, causing it to expand. If you go this route, though, be sure to get one that's adjustable, and take it off as soon as you're done having sex. You don't want to restrict bloodflow indefinitely.

▶ You'll have more energy. Stretching increases circulation. Better bloodflow means better erections and higher arousal levels. It can also improve your ability to take in oxygen and blow out carbon dioxide. Better breathing, as you learned on page 96, can even be the key to overcoming too-quick ejaculation.

▶ Regular stretching keeps muscles in balance, so that bones and joints are properly aligned. It's especially good for the "sexual core" muscles in the pelvis, hips, and abdomen— muscles that don't get much of a workout in an average day but are essential for comfortable and erotically charged moments.

It should be obvious by now that the benefits of stretching are hardly limited to the health club and that they extend beyond how you feel at any given moment. "When people stretch together, they become aware of each other's physical dimensions," says Paul Frediani, a personal trainer and former Golden Gloves champion. "Flexibility results in more freedom of movement during sex."

And that's the bottom line. Stretching will help you take sex to another level. Think of your favorite position. Now, imagine doing it with more flexibility and strength, with calmer nerves, greater vitality, and enhanced erotic energy. That's a whole lot of benefit from something that can take less time than wrestling with a tough condom wrapper.

## SEXUAL GAIN WITHOUT PAIN

Sex is about pleasure. Pleasure usually means an absence of pain. A simple equation—but judging from the comments we got when researching this book, a lot of us haven't quite figured it out.

Consider this note from a 45-year-old certified public accountant: *"I find that as I get older, some positions can become uncomfortable after a length of time, and a muscle cramp can be very distracting."*

Or this one from a 24-year-old IT support specialist: *"I pulled a leg muscle once trying an awkward position."* And this from an 18-year-old college student: *"I feel like I'm about to pull a groin muscle when I have sex."* Then there's this from a 42-year-old insurance rep: *"I threw my back out during sex."*

What's going on here? These guys are in the primes of their lives, for gawd's sake! If you're having this kind of pain during sex when you're 18 or 24 or 42, can you imagine what whoopee's going to be like when you're 50 or 60?

▼

**Surveys reveal that 98 percent of men would gladly increase the size of their penises if they knew a safe way to do it.**

▲

You're a lot more likely to avoid the sorts of aches and pains, and in some cases out-and-out injuries, that can take you out of service between the sheets just by maintaining a supple body. Studies show that most men don't stretch at all during the day. Without a little prep work prior to penetration, you can bet that their sexual horizons are a lot more limited than they need to be.

In fact, some sex books advise men to literally take a few minutes in the bedroom for some pre-sex stretching. Imagine the look on your partner's face when you say, "Excuse me, Honey"—then drop down on the carpet for some kind of Richard Simmons routine. *She'd* be the one getting cramps—from laughing so hard.

Not that some gentle stretching before sex is such a bad idea. But what you really need to be doing, and what makes a lot more sense in real life, is to set aside stretch time throughout the day. Timing doesn't matter very much. Muscles have memory: The stretching that you do in the morning or on your lunch break will pay off hours later when the lights go down.

But you have to stretch smart. You might think of stretching as "exercise lite," but if you do it without a little warmup and preparation, you aren't going to get limber, and you emphatically won't have better sex. Why? Because you'll get hurt. Here's what you need to do instead.

**RAISE YOUR BODY TEMPERATURE.** Yes, you'll need to warm up before doing any stretch, even the easy ones. In fact, it's just as important to warm up before stretching as it is prior to hard-core running or lifting. A warmup does just that: It raises your body temperature. A cold human body, like unheated plastic, breaks down during movement if it isn't warmed to sufficient pliability.

So before you stretch, do some simple, light moves. Walk for a few minutes. Stride from room to room. Swing your arms or do high knee lifts. Rotate your legs, your hips, your arms. A few minutes is enough. A rule of thumb: If you *feel* warm, you're warm enough to start stretching.

**FIGURE OUT WHAT YOU'RE DOING.** *Duh,* you say. But you'd be amazed how many men don't know how to stretch. They wind up doing the same moves—usually the wrong ones—that they see other guys doing at the gym. Think about this for a moment. How many of those guys would you trust to give authoritative advice on cardiovascular surgery or accounting or legal ways to keep the couch during a messy divorce? The ability to bench 280 pounds doesn't confer knowledge. When you stretch wrong, you can actually tear muscle fiber. Torn muscles can leave behind tough scar tissue that can elevate pain and stiffness to levels you don't want to contemplate.

At the very least, take the time to read some fitness books (including this one) and look closely at the stretching illustrations and instructions. Better yet, set up a meeting with a trainer. Most gyms include a session or two as part of the cost of membership. The benefits of smart stretching aren't limited to injury prevention. You'll probably wind up saving time as well because you'll learn how to get the most efficiency from each move.

**MAKE THE COMMITMENT.** Sorry, stretching isn't like winning the lottery. You have to keep punching your ticket, or you'll wind up like the Tin Man without WD-40. The only way you'll stay flexible is to keep working at it. You brush your teeth every day. Stretching deserves the same commitment, especially when you consider the erotic payoffs.

**DUMP THE TYPE A**. This is the hardest message to get across. Muscle work, like it or not, takes time. You can plan on stretching for at least a week before you'll notice any real difference in how you move. After that, it will be at least a month, and probably more, before you achieve anything resembling maximum flexibility—and before you fully reach your erotic potential.

## STRETCHING SMART

Stretching is typically divided into two types: static and ballistic. You can pretty much forget about the latter. It requires you to bob or bounce while performing some activity, like touching your toes. This type of stretching forcibly stretches a muscle, using your own momentum to hyperextend the muscle beyond its normal limit.

These days, ballistic stretching is pretty much frowned upon, except possibly for gymnasts and ballerinas. Unless you're already in great shape and are planning to have sex on a trapeze, there's never a good reason to jerk a muscle beyond its usual range of motion. It won't improve your performance in bed, and you'll probably spend the rest of the week walking around like Groucho Marx.

Static stretches are a lot more useful and are less likely to send you to a chiropractor. In static stretches, the muscle is stretched only to the point where you start to feel a pull. The idea is to extend the muscle almost, but not quite, to the point of discomfort. Going farther than that will tear tiny muscle fibers, damaging the area that you're trying to loosen and strengthen.

A simple example of a static stretch is to sit on the floor with your legs extended and reach forward to grab your toes. No bouncing or jolting—just a slow, steady pull.

Regardless of the specific stretches that you actually do—we've included static stretching programs for beginning, intermediate, and advanced levels—you want to hold each one for about 30 seconds. Trainers used to advise men to hold stretches for only 5 to 15 seconds, but studies have since shown that isn't anywhere near long enough to extend the muscle. In fact, it's probably no better for flexibility than not stretching at all. So follow the 30-second rule. You'll actually save time because a stretch held for that long is about as efficient as it gets. Conversely, don't bother holding the stretch for longer. You might think you're getting extra benefit when you hold a stretch for a minute or more, but it doesn't seem to be any more effective than a 30-second stretch.

Stretching is fundamentally pretty easy stuff. You can do it in the privacy of your home. You don't have to pop for equipment, and you can do it just about anywhere. About the only caveat is to maintain good posture: neck relaxed; head held naturally and aligned with the spine; shoulders down and back; stomach in; and knees slightly bent, not locked.

But you do want to stretch consistently—at least two or three times a week. Start slowly, of course; don't bounce (save that for the bedroom); and breathe deeply and easily throughout. Do each stretch at least half a dozen times, and don't forget to hold it for the full 30 seconds. Stretching won't make you a sexual athlete overnight. What it will do is give you the physical ability to go wherever your sexiest fantasies take you. How's that for motivation?

STRETCHES

## PHASE 1 ▶

**THE STRETCHES INCLUDED HERE ARE INTENDED FOR THE GUY WHO ISN'T A HARD-CORE ATHLETE**—who wants to gain flexibility and strength in bed while at the same time being better able to perform comfortably in just about any of the usual positions. Each of the stretches in this section will also increase power in the chest, arms, back, and legs. If you're spending time in the so-called missionary position, for example, these stretches will help ensure that you don't get crippled by cramps. At the same time, they'll strengthen and give flexibility to muscles in the lower back and abdomen—necessary for comfortable thrusting.

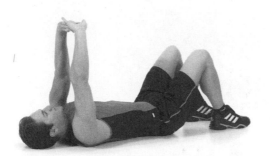

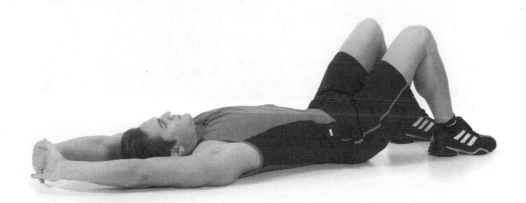

## SHOULDERS

Lie on your back and extend your arms above your shoulders, perpendicular to the floor. Clasp your fingers together with your palms facing the ceiling. Keeping your arms straight, slowly lower them until your hands rest on the floor behind your head. Hold for 30 seconds, return to the starting position, and repeat.

▶*Sexual Gains:* **This stretch enhances your stamina in man-on-top positions by easing the toll on your shoulders.**

## STRETCHES: PHASE 1

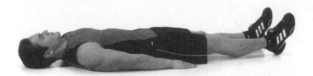

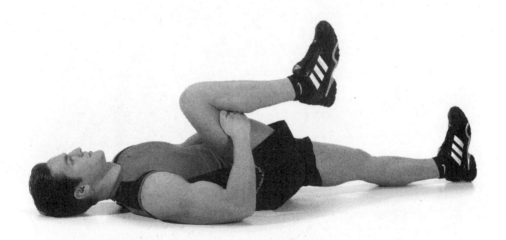

### HIPS

Lie on your back with your legs straight. Grasp your right upper thigh with both hands and pull your right knee toward your chest. Hold for 30 seconds, return to the starting position, then repeat. Do the same thing with your left leg.

▶*Sexual Gains:* **Stretching the hips allows you to thrust stronger and longer.**

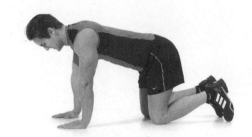

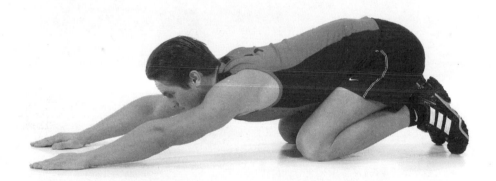

## LOWER BACK

Get on your hands and knees, with your hands directly under your shoulders. Keeping your hands in place, sit back on your heels until you feel a stretch along your back; your arms will be outstretched at this point. Hold for 30 seconds, then repeat.

▶*Sexual Gains:* **Improves endurance and strength for kneeling positions and standing positions when you're supporting most of her weight and yours.**

## STRETCHES: PHASE 1

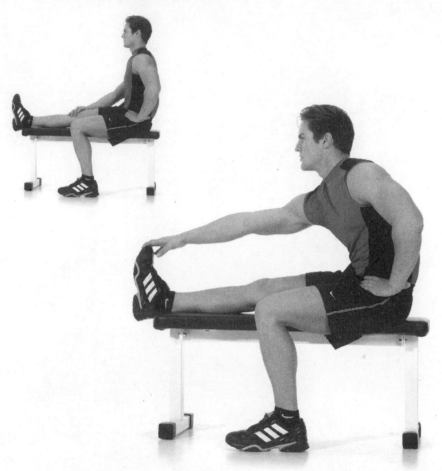

## HAMSTRINGS

Sit on the edge of a bed or bench. With your left foot on the floor, raise your right leg and extend it. Put your right hand on your right knee and slowly slide it forward until you touch your toes—or as close as you can comfortably get. Hold for 30 seconds. Then stretch the left leg.

▶*Sexual Gains:* **This exercise is better than similar stretches in which you sit on the floor because it puts less strain on the lower back. Flexible hamstrings improve your endurance and strength in standing and kneeling positions.**

STRETCHES: PHASE **1**

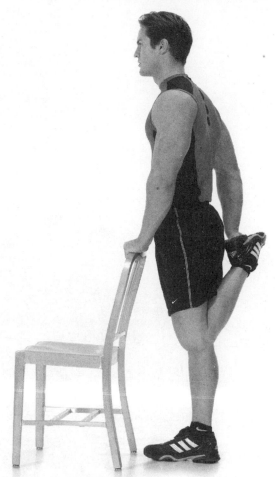

## THIGHS

Stand, resting your left hand on a wall or the back of a chair for
support. Bend your left knee and grab your left foot with your right
hand. Pull your foot up until the heel presses against your butt.
Hold for 30 seconds. Repeat with the right leg.

▶*Sexual Gains:* **Flexibility in the front of the thigh
(quadriceps) will help you kneel for long periods and counter-
push when she's on top.**

STRETCHES: PHASE 1

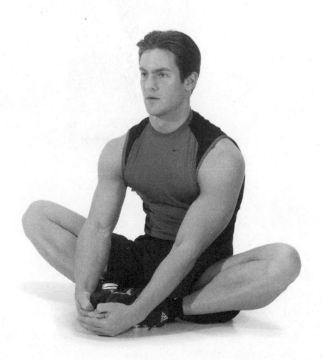

## GROIN

Sit on the floor with your back straight. Draw your feet up to your body until the soles touch. Let your knees drop to either side, but don't overextend the muscles by letting them drop too far. Hold for 30 seconds, then repeat.

▶*Sexual Gains:* **Stretching the groin area allows for stronger thrusting and greater versatility in positioning.**

STRETCHES: PHASE 1

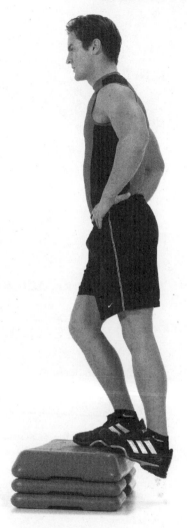

## CALVES

Stand on a step and lower the heel of your left foot over the edge of the step until you feel a tug. Hold for 30 seconds. Repeat with your right foot.

▶*Sexual Gains:* **This stretch prevents the crippling cramps men sometimes experience from overflexing their calves during orgasm.**

STRETCHES

# PHASE 2 ▶

**LET'S ASSUME THAT YOU WORK OUT A LOT. MAYBE YOU RUN OR SWIM A FEW TIMES A WEEK OR LIFT WEIGHTS PRETTY REGULARLY.** Or you've been doing the Phase 1 stretches for several weeks, and they are starting to seem easy and effortless. These stretches are a little bit harder than the ones in Phase 1, with a correspondingly greater payoff: You might find yourself attempting some sexual positions you haven't tried before—holding your partner and having sex while standing, to name just one tempting example.

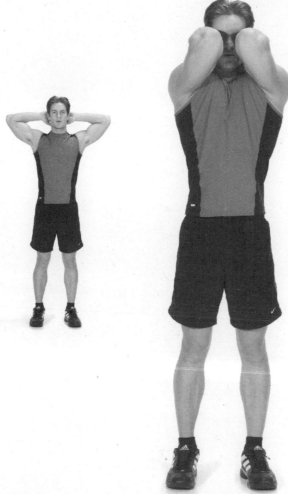

## CHEST

Clasp your hands behind your head, with your elbows out to the sides. Inhale and exhale naturally while moving your elbows in front of your face. Hold the stretch, then move your elbows to the sides until you feel a stretch in your chest. Hold for 30 seconds, then repeat.

▶*Sexual Gains:* **Improves breathing capacity; helps you last longer when you're on top or during rear-entry sex when you're supporting yourself with your arms.**

STRETCHES: PHASE 2

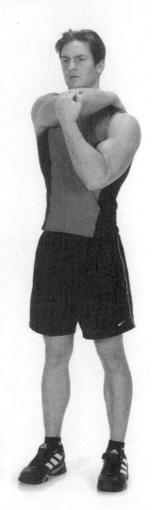

## SHOULDERS

Grab the back of your right elbow with your left hand. Pull your
right arm across your body and up and under your chin—or at least
as far as you comfortably can. Hold for 30 seconds. Repeat with
the left arm.

▶*Sexual Gains:* **Gives you better range of motion for
reaching around and caressing your partner in positions where
you're behind her.**

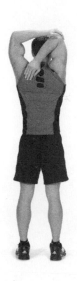
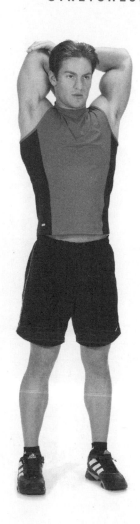

## TRICEPS

Lift your right arm over your head and, with your left hand, gently push back on the right triceps, just above your elbow. Hold for 30 seconds, then repeat with the left arm.

▶*Sexual Gains:* **Improves arm stamina during man-on-top sex and while performing manual stimulation.**

STRETCHES: PHASE **2**

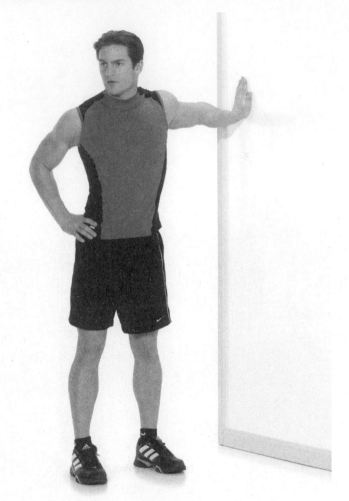

## BICEPS

Rest your left hand against a wall. Turn your torso away from the wall and extend your arm as straight as you can, until you feel a stretch in the left biceps. Hold for 30 seconds. Repeat with the right arm.

▶*Sexual Gains:* **Improves endurance in standing and other positions when you're supporting her weight with your arms, and when performing manual stimulation.**

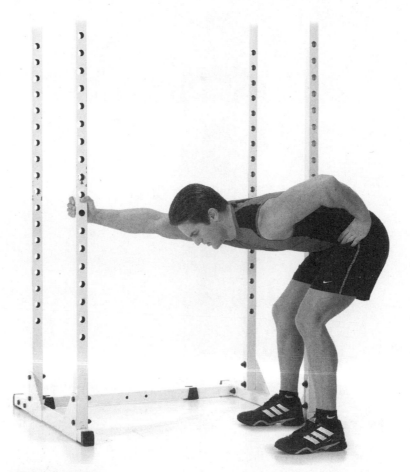

## UPPER BACK

Find a sturdy bar (or a horizontal surface that's about chest high). Stand about 3 feet away from it, bend at the waist, lean forward, and grip the bar with your right hand. Lower your head and chest until you feel a good stretch in your upper back. Hold for 30 seconds, then switch arms and repeat.

▶ *Sexual Gains:* **Improves endurance and flexibility in man-on-top positions and seated positions when you're leaning forward, holding her up.**

STRETCHES: PHASE 2

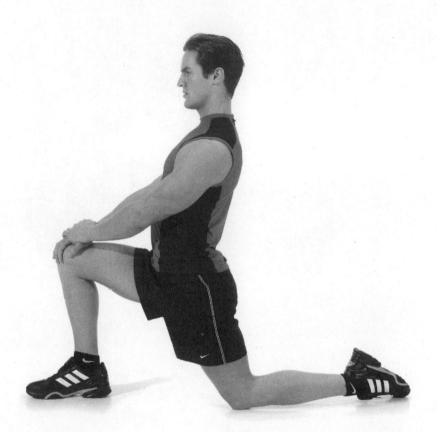

## THIGHS

Kneel on your left knee with your right foot about 2 feet in front of you. Tilt your pelvis forward by tucking your glutes under your torso and pulling your belly button toward your spine. Place both hands on your right knee, then shift your body weight forward until you feel a stretch in the top of your left thigh. Hold for 30 seconds. Repeat with the left leg.

▶*Sexual Gains:* **Allows better range of motion in sitting and kneeling positions.**

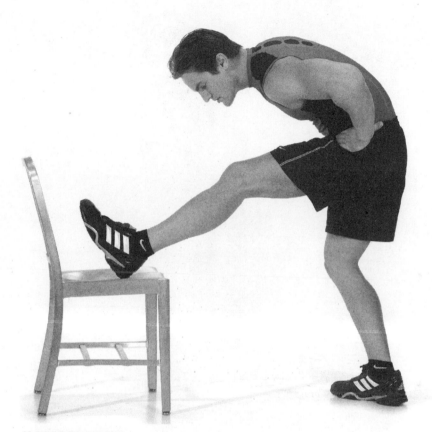

## HAMSTRINGS

Rest your left foot on a chair and bend your torso over your leg as if you're trying to touch your knee with your forehead. Keep the knee slightly bent. Hold the stretch for 30 seconds. Repeat with the right leg.

▶*Sexual Gains:* **Gives you better range of motion for positions in which you're behind your partner or you're both standing and leaning over a table or bed.**

STRETCHES: PHASE 2

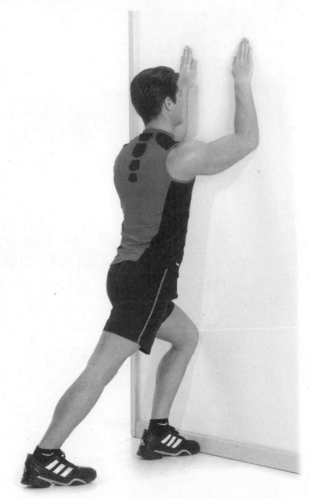

## CALVES

Stand facing a wall and rest your forearms on it. Move your right foot back 3 to 4 feet. Bend your left leg, keeping your right leg straight. Keeping your right heel on the floor, lean even closer to the wall, until you feel a good stretch in your right calf. Hold for 30 seconds. Repeat with the left leg.

▶*Sexual Gains:* **Improves your range of motion and endurance for subtle tiptoe thrusts in man-on-top positions.**

STRETCHES

# PHASE 3 ▶

**YOU WON'T HAVE A WHOLE LOT OF TROUBLE WITH THE STRETCHES WE'VE DISCUSSED SO FAR.** Now it's time for the next phase of the program, one that can push your muscles—and the sexual activity you'll use them for—into the stratosphere. Once again, each of these stretches focuses on the muscles you use most during sex. When you get through this program, you'll have flexibility you never dreamed of, along with more energy and a lot more sexual endurance.

Obviously, you don't want to attempt this program until you're already in good shape—at a minimum, after several weeks of doing the easier stretches.

STRETCHES: PHASE 3

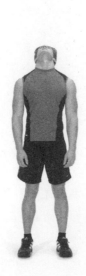

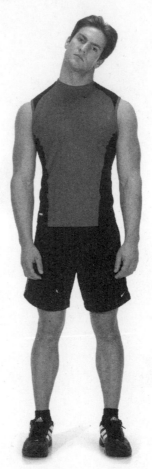

## NECK

Relax your shoulders and drop your chin to your chest. Let it hang there for about 30 seconds. Raise your head slowly to an upright position and keep going, until you're looking at the ceiling. Hold it for 30 seconds, then return your head to level. Next, tilt your head so that your left ear moves toward your left shoulder. Keep your shoulders still. Hold the stretch for about 30 seconds, then slowly raise your head and repeat on the right side.

▶ *Sexual Gains:* **Prevents neck and shoulder cramps and allows for greater range of motion when you're performing oral sex.**

STRETCHES: PHASE **3**

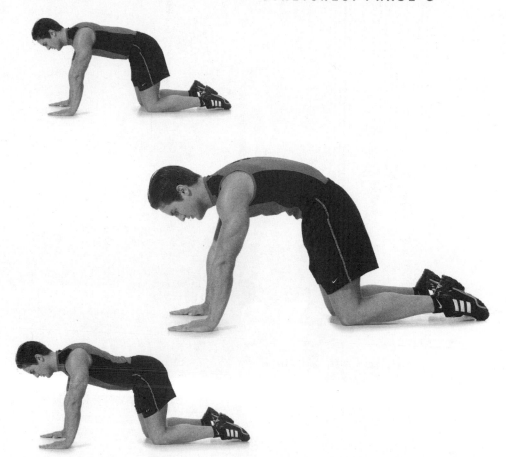

## BACK

Get down on your hands and knees, with your back straight. Arch your back as high as you comfortably can. Hold for 30 seconds, then relax and repeat. Next, lower your belly, dropping your back as low as you comfortably can. Relax and repeat.

▶*Sexual Gains:* **Improves range of motion and endurance for mutual oral sex positions.**

STRETCHES: PHASE 3

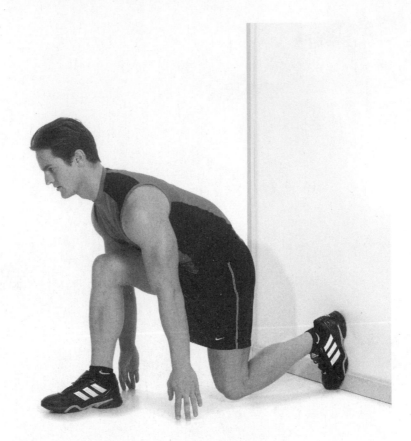

## HIPS

Stand with your back about 2 feet from a wall. Extend your left leg behind you and press the heel against the wall. Bend your right knee and squat until your right thigh is parallel to the floor. Your right knee should be directly over your heel, so that your shin is at a 90-degree angle to the floor. Resting your fingertips lightly on the floor to keep yourself steady, press your left heel firmly into the wall, straightening your left leg while tightening the thigh muscles. Hold for 30 seconds. Repeat with the other foot.

▶*Sexual Gains*: **Improves hip-flexor range of motion so you can arch your back for maximum penetration.**

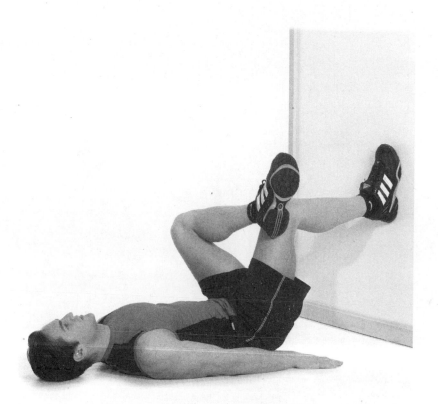

## BUTT

Lie on your back, with your knees bent. Put your right foot on a wall, with the shin parallel to the floor. Place your left foot on your right thigh near the knee. (If the bottom of your spine lifts off the floor, move away from the wall until it rests firmly on the floor.) Hold the stretch for 30 seconds. Repeat with the other foot.

▶*Sexual Gains:* **Improves hip motion during thrusting.**

## STRETCHES: PHASE 3

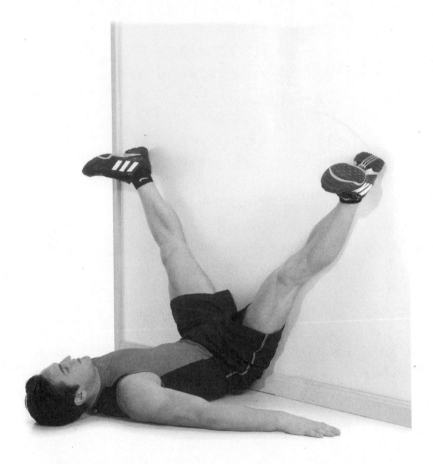

## THIGHS

Lie on your back and extend your legs up a wall. With the back of your pelvis flat on the floor and your glutes resting against the wall, allow your legs to open slowly. Go as far as you comfortably can. Press the backs of your knees and legs against the wall. Let the full weight of your torso relax downward. If your knees hurt, bring your legs closer together. Hold the stretch for 30 seconds, then repeat.

▶*Sexual Gains:* **Increases stamina and range of motion in kneeling and standing positions.**

# STRETCHING FOR TWO ▶

**THINK THAT EXERCISE ISN'T FUN? OH, HOW WRONG YOU ARE**—when you exercise (maybe that should be "sexercise") with your partner. There's certainly potential for fun, especially when there's a good chance that the workout will wind up in bed.

The following stretching exercises are effective and reasonably easy for just about everyone. We picked them specifically because they lend themselves to increased flexibility in bed. At the same time, they'll give you and your partner something to think about, and who knows where that might lead?

Here's the thing: When you stretch with a partner, it's almost impossible not to talk about the experience. You need to tell each other when a stretch is too much or too little; you'll also find yourself talking about what you're feeling at the moment, physically as well as emotionally. You don't need 17 sessions in couples' counseling to know that the more you express your particular needs, the sexier you're likely to feel. Talk during exercise naturally leads to talk about sex, not to mention talk during sex. That can get pretty hot indeed.

Of course, watching your partner move in exercise is enticing in its own right. Mutual stretching allows you to be intimate with one another without being sexual. Think of it as a kind of extended foreplay.

The key to partner exercise is communication. Let each other know how far to stretch and when to stop. As always, move slowly and with total control, without bouncing or straining. Ease into each stretch. Relax. Enjoy.

STRETCHES: STRETCHING FOR TWO

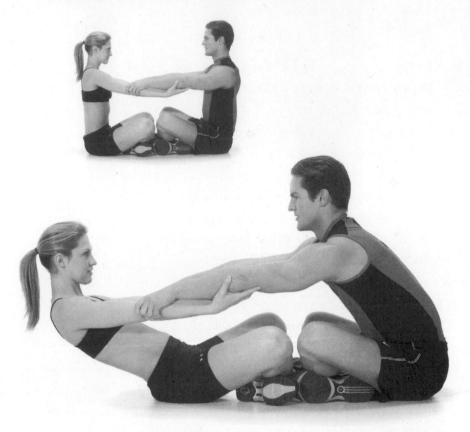

## PULL IT TOGETHER

Sit on the floor facing your partner. Each of you should have your legs crossed, with your knees nearly touching. Grip each other's forearms in a way that is comfortable and allows you both to sit up straight. Lean back slowly, gently bringing your partner toward you. Be sure to keep your butt planted on the floor. Next, your partner takes the lead, repeating the stretch. Hold each stretch for 30 seconds, then return to an upright position. Repeat five or six times.

▶ *Sexual Gains:* **Stretches the hips, lower back, and shoulders, which improves endurance during seated sex, when backs and shoulders tend to cramp and fatigue.**

STRETCHES: STRETCHING FOR TWO

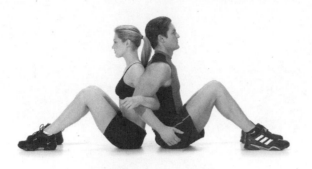

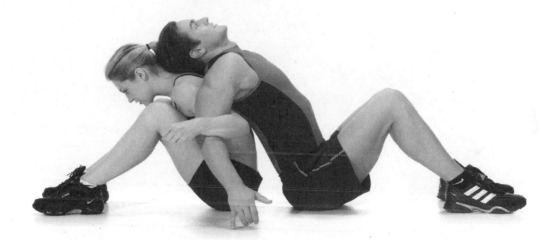

## BACK TO BACK

Sit on the floor back to back. Your knees should be bent and relaxed, with your feet flat on the floor. Interlock your elbows with your partner's. Slowly lean forward, bringing your head toward your knees. Your partner should relax and allow herself to stretch back with you as far as is comfortable. Slowly return to an upright position. Next, your partner takes the lead, repeating the movements by leaning forward. Repeat five or six times, holding each stretch for 30 seconds.

▶*Sexual Gains:* **Flexes the back muscles, allowing you to lean off the edge of the bed and say, "Ahh."**

STRETCHES: STRETCHING FOR TWO

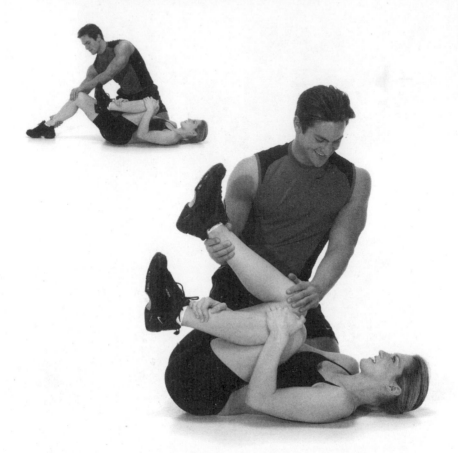

## HIP FLEX

Lie on your back, with your right leg bent and your right foot flat on the floor. Your partner kneels on the floor at your right side. Grab your left knee and ankle with both hands. Your partner, meanwhile, holds your right knee and ankle, gently stretching the knee toward your chest while keeping the ankle in line with the knee. Exchange places with your partner. Hold this position for 30 seconds, then switch legs and repeat the stretch. Repeat two or three times.

▶*Sexual Gains:* **Maximizes your thrusting power and allows her to extend her legs all the way up and back for the deepest penetration.**

**STRETCHES: STRETCHING FOR TWO**

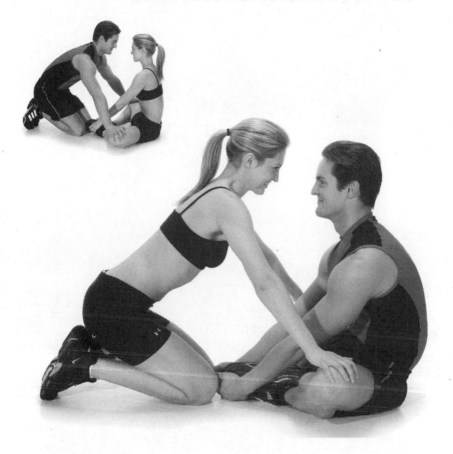

## KNEE PRESS

Your partner should sit on the floor, with the soles of her feet together and her knees bent. Facing her, place your hands on her knees, and *gently* press them toward the floor. Then switch positions and let her take over. Hold each stretch for 30 seconds, then relax. Repeat five or six times.

▶*Sexual Gains:* **Stretches the inner thighs, improving comfort during sitting positions and range of motion for her to wrap her legs around you.**

STRETCHES: STRETCHING FOR TWO

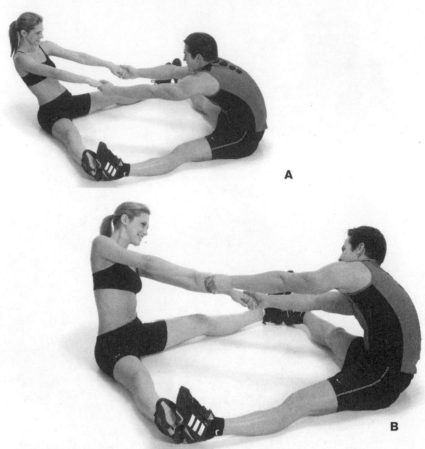

A

B

## THE DIAMOND

Sit on the floor facing one another, with your legs extended in a
comfortable V-shape. Press the bottoms of your feet against the
bottoms of your partner's feet. Reach out and grip each other's
hands. Next, while holding hands, have your partner slowly and
gently lean forward, hold for a few seconds, then lean back. You, of
course, follow.

Depending on your respective heights and your initial degree of
flexibility, you may not be able to move more than an inch or two,
but you will definitely feel the stretch in the back of your legs. After
a bit, try leaning to the right, holding for a few seconds, then leaning

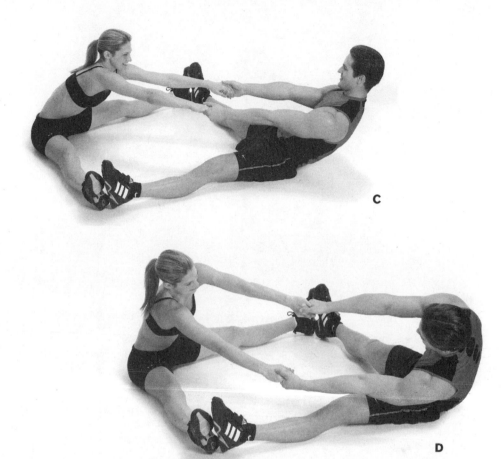

C

D

to the left. Next, try a circle: lean forward (A), to the right (B), back (C), and to the left (D). Keep going.

Take this one slowly and gently, until you've both achieved some flexibility. And don't push it: The stretch becomes counterproductive if you cause pain in the person with the shorter legs.

▶*Sexual Gains:* **Stretches the hamstrings, inner thighs, and calves, providing better endurance and range of motion in standing, kneeling, and sitting positions.**

**STRETCHES: STRETCHING FOR TWO**

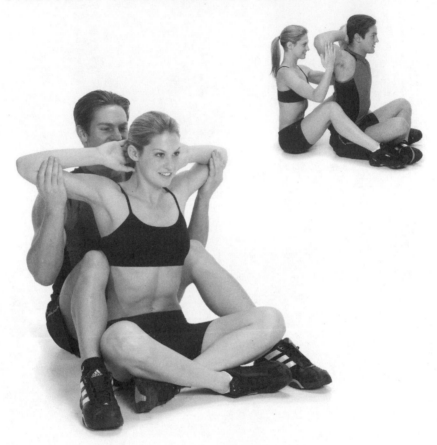

## THE BUTTERFLY

Your partner should sit cross-legged on the floor, with her hands behind her head and her elbows out to the sides. You sit behind her, with your legs on either side of hers. Place your hands on her arms just above her elbows. Next, *gently* pull her elbows back toward you, until she feels a stretch across her chest. Don't pull too hard or too fast. Then it's her turn to stretch you. Hold each stretch for 30 seconds. Repeat several times.

▶ *Sexual Gains:* **Improves range of motion and comfort when switching from one position to another or when you get adventurous with silk scarves and bedposts.**

STRETCHES: STRETCHING FOR TWO

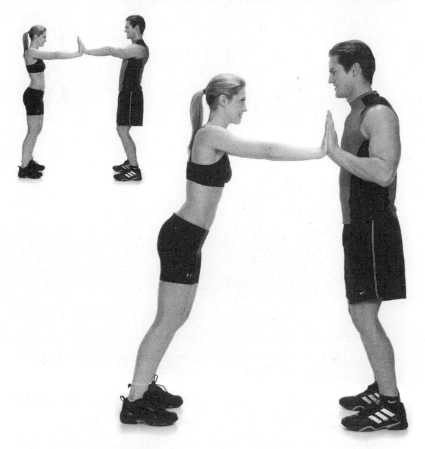

## SHOULDER PRESS

Stand face to face with your partner. Your feet should be shoulder-width apart and your knees slightly bent. Extend your arms in front so that your palms touch and your fingers point to the ceiling. Have your partner bend her elbows, easing you toward her. Hold for about 10 seconds, or as long as is comfortable. She then pushes you back to the upright position and leans toward you. Try 10 to 20 times in each direction.

▶*Sexual Gains:* **Stretches the shoulders and arms, allowing each of you to reach down with ease for manual stimulation during foreplay and intercourse.**

# CHAPTER 6

# THE *BUILT*
# *FOR SEX* WORKOUT

**NEWS FLASH: WOMEN APPRECIATE MEN WITH GOOD PHYSIQUES JUST AS MUCH AS MEN ENJOY FIT WOMEN. IMAGINE THAT.**

Men will always be more visually inclined than women, and you can thank your lucky stars for that. Very few of the women we talked to listed Stallone-like muscles at the top of their wish lists. In fact, they're far less likely than men to reject a potential suitor because he's in less-than-perfect shape. But do they appreciate a well-toned body? You bet.

*"A muscular upper body and strong arms are a real turn-on,"* said a 41-year-old hospital administrator in Buffalo. *"I love toned legs, when you can see the outline of his calf and quad muscles,"* said a 33-year-old Portland, Oregon, biologist. And this from a 37-year-old medical student in Albuquerque: *"Some men have a great chest or a nice butt that you just want to get your hands on. But that doesn't mean he has to be 6 feet tall or as strong as an ox."*

If nothing else, it's worth staying in shape—or getting there if you haven't yet made the commitment to buckle down in the gym—just to make yourself more attractive to a current or future partner. The benefits don't stop there. Men who stay in shape have more energy. More energy for sex, for working, for life in general. Exercise makes you happier and more self-assured. Most important, it improves the machinery—bloodflow, nerve activity, and brain chemistry, for example—that you need for full-bore sex appeal and performance.

## FIT FOR LOVE

How strong do you have to be for sex? Stronger than you might think—unless your idea of passionate coupling is to imitate one of the stiffs on *CSI*. Even when you're in the passive, man-on-the-bottom position, you need strong abs and hips to push your body upward. Men who are really out of shape often find themselves getting fatigued before the act is done—as well as sore the next day. That's not very sexy. Or satisfying. And that's an *easy* position. How are you going to feel when you try something more athletic?

If you plan on doing anything more vigorous than just lying there during sex, you're going to need strength, flexibility, and endurance. Consider the man-on-top position. You need a strong chest and strong arms to move with any kind of freedom as well as to hold your weight off your partner. Sex while standing? You'd better have some muscles in your calves, hamstrings, and butt.

*"When I'm on top, I find it hard to hold myself up for long periods of time,"* admits a 21-year-old student in Pittsburgh. *"With all the thrusting and whatnot, my back and abs seem to give out sooner than I'd like."*

The doctors we talked to said that this guy's story is hardly unique. Even though men are more health conscious today than they've ever been, that doesn't always translate into committed workouts. Basically, we spend way too much time at our desks, sitting in our cars, and taking up couch space. Our sex lives are paying the price. Even our *desire* for sex may be heading downhill.

It's not news to exercise physiologists that men who are sedentary can have significant drops in testosterone, the "male" hormone that fuels libido. Add to that the natural drop in testosterone that occurs when men get older, and you can see why a lot of us aren't exactly thrilled with our bedroom oomph.

None of this is inevitable. The amount of exercise that you need for optimal sexual fitness is modest. Half an hour or so in the gym most days of the week will give you endurance, energy, and sex drive that you didn't even know you had. Harder workouts, if you're so inclined, can boost your performance even more. Finnish researchers recently reported that 30-year-old men who engaged in regular weight lifting had significant boosts in testosterone. More testosterone quickly translates to more muscle bulk, faster recovery after workouts, and in some cases, a boost in libido.

*"I'm living proof,"* a 23-year-old student in Boston told us. *"I lost 80 pounds and started lifting. I now have more sex and better sex for longer periods, with no next-day soreness."*

Better sex by itself should be reason enough to strive for the exercise edge. But it's not the only reason.

▶ Men who lift weights get *more* limber, not less. Your balance will improve as well.

▶ Strength training increases bone strength and density. That means less risk of fractures.

▶ It "oils" the joints and lowers the risk of arthritis. It makes it easier to ski, run, or just get around in this world without bum joints.

▸ It increases the level of beneficial HDL cholesterol, which carts the artery-clogging stuff out of your bloodstream before it lays down rock-hard deposits in the arteries that supply the penis.

▸ Men who start a strength-training program invariably report a huge increase in confidence—the quality that nearly all women rate at the top of their sex-appeal charts.

Whether you're interested mainly in building muscle, strengthening bones, or increasing sexual stamina, lifting weights should be your first choice. Muscles grow only in response to high-intensity over-load—pumping iron, in other words. Moving your arms up and

## ATHLETES AND ABSTINENCE

When the Los Angeles Dodgers struggled early in the 2003 season, more than a few commentators floated the suggestion that their performance might improve if players took a little break from their, er, marital arrangements. None of the players actually volunteered (publicly, at least) to "give it up" for the team, and the Dodgers eventually found their footing and made the playoffs anyway.

This story is a perfect illustration of the widespread belief that athletes who have sex before competing somehow lose their edge. The myth persists even though scientific studies—yes, researchers have studied it—clearly show that having sex in no way diminishes an athlete's performance. One study tested the grip strength of married athletes, ages 24 to 49, the morning after intercourse and the morning after abstinence. There were no differences in grip strength on either morning. A few years later, another study looked at grip strength plus aerobic capacity and coordination. Again, sex the night before made no difference. In fact, some research suggests that athletes actually perform better when they roll in the hay before they play.

down all day won't do a thing for bulk or strength. But put something heavy in your hands, and if that something is heavier than what your arms are accustomed to, you're going to get stronger.

## MORE OF WHAT YOU ARE

If you're new to the health-club scene, check your ego at the door. It doesn't matter if you're burly, skinny, tanned, or pale—your physique isn't going to match up to the guys who are clustered around dumbbells the size of Volkswagens. More than a few men walk into the gym and instantly "compare and despair"—and give up because they're too self-conscious to work out next to men who look like they move refrigerators all day.

If you really want to make yourself feel better, remind yourself that (1) a lot of those guys have been lifting for years, (2) the real-life monsters among them have probably been blasting steroids, and (3) all of those black-market drugs are inexorably wrecking them with acne, liver damage, and impotence—and reducing their testicles to the size of peanuts.

Trainers are used to men who come in the door with visions of tree-trunk thighs and anaconda arms filling their heads. Sure, you could be the next Mr. Universe, but that has less to do with commitment than with your basic physical makeup. A strength-training program can make you more of what you already are; it won't transform you into something you're not. A tall, thin man isn't going to emerge a year later with a neck like Mike Tyson's, any more than a short, stocky guy is going to get whippet lean.

And that's a good thing. Research backs up what the women we surveyed said. Yes, they like physical fitness and good muscle tone, but chances are they're looking for a regular guy—not the guy grinning at you from the cover of a body-building magazine. Two studies from the University of Texas in Austin found that women preferred men with waist-to-hip ratios in the normal range. Sure, that means John Goodman wouldn't make their "hotties" list, but neither would Arnold Schwarzenegger.

Lifting weights will definitely improve your health. It will probably boost your libido and your ability to sustain erections. What it won't do is overturn your basic genetic structure. Ever wonder why so many bench-press champs are stubby little guys with short arms? They were born with short bones, which give them great leverage. Anyone who lifts regularly will get bigger and stronger. The extent to which you bulk up has a lot to do with the genes that nature gave you.

Consider your muscle makeup. All men possess a combination of fast-twitch and slow-twitch muscles. Men with a greater percentage of slow-twitch muscles are better suited to aerobic exercise (think distance runners); they'll have a hard time adding much muscle mass. Those with an edge in fast-twitch fibers put on muscle and gain strength more easily—and tend to accumulate body fat more quickly (think power lifters). You can't change your basic muscle equation. The percentage of fast- and slow-twitch fibers that you're born with is the percentage you'll keep.

Age also plays a role in how quickly you'll advance. A man's testosterone levels rise sharply in his second decade of life and continue rising at a slower pace until about age 30. All of that testosterone makes it easy to add muscle mass. Once you're in your 40s, though, you have to work harder to get the same effect.

Researchers in the world of exercise science spend their whole careers studying the finer points of weight lifting. For the most part, though, it pretty much boils down to this: Pick it up, put it down, pick it up again. There isn't a whole lot more to it than that. Of course, there is a handful of training tips that you'll want to keep in mind.

**START WITH THE 8-WEEK RULE.** If you're just starting out, you'll want to stick with the same basic program—these exercises for your biceps, those for your chest, and so on—for about 8 weeks. That's about how long it takes to kick your muscles into gear and prime your body. It also takes about that long to lock yourself into the habit of exercise.

**SHAKE IT UP IN TWO.** A lot of experienced lifters find themselves in an exercise rut. They do the same exercises and keep doing them, month after month. There are two problems with this approach. This first is tedium; doing the same exercises again and again is about as exciting as brushing your teeth. More important, muscles need change to keep growing. Sure, you'll keep getting stronger if you do the same workouts, but after about 8 weeks, the gains start to accrue at a snail's pace. You'll get more improvements

## I LOVE YOU, SUE . . . ER, CINDY

Plenty of men having sex with one woman fill their heads with fantasies about someone else, and plenty of women do the same. Most of the time, the fantasies never make the injudicious journey from the brain to the mouth—which is a good thing, because no one wants to be called by the wrong name during moments of passion.

Is it a kind of mental infidelity to think of someone else during sex? Some women (and men) think it is. Researchers, on the other hand, say that nearly everyone does it on occasion. In most of these cases, the fantasies that occur during sex are no different from any other fantasies: They can stir your sense of eroticism without ever crossing over into reality.

There is one difference, though. In general, sharing fantasies with your partner can bring the two of you closer, but admitting that you're thinking of someone else altogether probably isn't the smartest thing to do.

Of course, all sorts of things can slip out in the heat of the moment. Which is why more than a few wise lovers never use their partners' names during sex. Generic terms of endearment—"Oh, Baby"—work just as well and minimize the possibility of mistakes.

more quickly if you vary your workouts—adding new exercises, subtracting old ones, or adding twists and refinements—about every 2 weeks. The idea is to avoid training plateaus—those dead zones where further improvement virtually stops.

**WORK HARD, REST HARDER.** As long as men have been lifting weights, trainers have been arguing about the optimal amount of downtime. These days, the usual advice for regular guys is to lift 3 days a week—every other day, for example—and rest in between. Men in their 20s or 30s who are already in great shape might do better with four weekly workouts. Unless you're a competitive athlete, it's highly unlikely that working out more often will provide extra benefits. If anything, it will increase your risk of injury.

Rest is important for another reason. You might think that your muscles get larger while you're lifting, but that's not what happens. When you're at the gym, you're actually tearing down muscle fibers. The growth phase occurs when muscles repair themselves—and that happens only *after* you leave the gym.

## FIND A CLUB THAT WORKS

Most men have tried lifting weights at one time or another. Most have signed up at a health club. And most stick with it—until they find something more interesting to do, like setting up a home entertainment system.

Why do so many good intentions get derailed? Part of it is habit. It takes about 6 weeks before any new activity stops feeling new and becomes just another part of your life, like pulling on your socks every morning. It's also because your whole body rebels when you're out of shape. Start pushing those tired, locked-tight muscles farther than they're used to going, and they're going to fight back. Almost no one enjoys working out for the first week or two. At best, it seems boring—and at worst, it hurts.

You have to push through that initial despair zone. Finding a good club is the best way to do it. Here's what experts advise.

**PUT CONVENIENCE FIRST.** Just about every city has at least a few health clubs that resemble opulent palaces, replete with fresh towels, the latest glistening chrome, and glass-walled aerobics rooms to facilitate women-watching. They're great places to hang out. They're even great places to work out. But if they aren't located in an area that's near your home or office—or somewhere in between—you'll find all sorts of reasons not to bother. The best gym, even if it's a sweat-stained cave with flickering fluorescent lights that haven't been changed since the Carter Administration, is the one that's easiest to get to.

**CHECK OUT THE INVENTORY.** Health clubs have taken a hint from big-box shopping centers: warehouse-size spaces with an abundance of benches, free weights, and machines. It's a good approach. Even if you like the cozy atmosphere of an intimate, small-scale club, the last thing you want is to come in all fired up and then spend 20 minutes or so bored out of your nut because clots of muscle-heads won't budge from the machines. Before you sign on the dotted line, drop by the club a few times at the hours you're most likely to go. You should be able to launch into your workout without having to wait more than a few minutes to get to a weight bench or machine.

**SCHEDULE A SESSION.** Nearly all health clubs offer one or two consultations with a trainer as part of the sign-up cost. Take advantage of it. If you're totally new to lifting, you'll want to get solid instruction on using the equipment, honing your technique, and not getting hurt. Even if you've been lifting for years, a trainer can help correct bad habits and mistakes that you've unconsciously slipped into.

**KNOW THE RAP ON REPS.** Lifting, like any specialized activity, has its share of jargon. About all you really need to know is the difference between reps and sets.

*Rep* is short for repetition. If you lift a weight eight consecutive times, you've done eight reps. Sets are groups of repetitions—for example, three sets of eight repetitions.

Once you know that, the rest is mostly details—details that, for the average guy, won't make a whit of difference. It's true that doing multiple sets adds bulk to muscles more quickly than doing single sets. Some trainers swear that you're better off doing a single set of all-out exercises, heaving the maximum weight you can manage. Others argue for doing multiple sets of lesser intensity. Don't worry about it. If your schedule permits, by all means take the time to do multiple sets. If time is short, make do with singles. All of the refinements are mainly for guys who take the whole thing way too seriously. Let's face it, if you haven't done a lot of lifting in the past, any kind of lifting is going to make a difference. You can always refine your workout later.

**LIFT FOR TWO, RELAX FOR FOUR.** There's no such thing as speed lifting, not that you'd know it from watching the supermacho, muscle-packed dudes who turn every lifting move into something that sounds like a bus smash. They heave up impossibly huge weights, then let them come crashing down. It's all posturing. For one thing, lowering weights too quickly reduces muscle-building strain on the muscles. It's also a great way to get hurt. The fact is, those guys could probably cut the weights in half and get the same or better workouts if they took their time and used good form.

The fastest way to build muscle is to lift and lower weights with total control. The idea is to let your muscles, not gravity, guide each move. You want to complete the exertion phase in a count of two and the relaxing phase in a count of four. Don't obsess over the numbers, though. The most important thing is to lift naturally, without heaving and grunting—or letting go at the end.

**KEEP PUSHING.** The only way you'll develop bigger, stronger muscles is to work with progressively heavier weights. Once you're able to complete, say, eight repetitions at a given weight, it's time to bump up the weight. Research has shown that beginners usually do best when they start with a weight that's about 40 percent less than the maximum weight they could possibly handle. For example, if you can lift 100 pounds on the bench press when you go all out, start with 60 pounds. Stick with it for a week or two, or until it's clearly too easy. At that point, add more weight.

▼

**Men who lift weights regularly tend to have less acne than men who are sedentary. Reason: Sweating heavily during exercise, assuming you clean your skin thoroughly afterward, flushes the pores of acne-causing dirt and debris.**

▲

Start with a weight that allows you to do at least 8 reps. Once you can achieve 12 reps with that weight, increase it by about 5 percent. You'll then be doing 8 reps with the slightly heavier weight. Once you've worked up again to 12 reps with the heavier weight, step it up another 5 percent. The idea is to keep increasing, alternately, reps and resistance, so that you continue to achieve results.

The simplest way to figure out how much weight you should attempt on each exercise is through trial by ordeal. Pick up a weight and try eight reps. If you can't make eight, you need to select a lighter weight. Keep going until you've found a weight you can lift eight times, but not nine. The ideal weight should fatigue you by rep five but not actually wear you out until eight.

If your main goal is to improve cardiovascular endurance, you'll want to focus on doing more repetitions with lighter weights. For brute strength, you'll employ heavier weights in fewer repetitions. For overall muscle tone—the optimal place for beginners—lift medium weights, trying to complete 10 to 12 repetitions per set.

**SPLIT YOUR ROUTINES.** This simply means working different muscle groups on different days. Many lifters, for example, work their chests and backs on one day, then their legs and arms on the next. The advantage of this approach is that you get a more concentrated workout. At the same time, each muscle group gets a day off when you shift your focus to a different area. Over the course of two or three workouts, you hit all of your muscles—and then you start all over again.

You can split a routine in any number of ways.

▶ Divide your workouts into upper- and lower-body routines.

▶ Divide them into pushing and pulling exercises. Pushing exercises include squats and presses, while pulling movements include deadlifts, curls, rows, and pulldowns.

▶ Divide your body front to back. Most of the muscles on the front of your body, along with your calves and triceps, involve pushing exercises. The muscles on the back of your body, along with the biceps, usually involve pulling movements.

▶ Work the big muscles first. Time is limited. Energy is limited. And let's face it, your patience has limits as well. There will always be times when you drag yourself to the gym, do one or two sets of a few exercises, then make a sudden detour to the hot tub. To ensure that you can get some sort of workout every time you go, focus on the big muscles first: the thighs, chest, and so on. Save the small-muscle workouts, like those focusing on the wrists or triceps, for the last part of the workout. Even if you bail early, the big-muscle exercises will have hit most of the minor muscles as well.

## SEX-SPECIFIC STRENGTH TRAINING

There are all sorts of reasons men lift weights. The main ones are to look better and feel better, and that's about as good as motivation gets. But in the following pages, we've done something a little different. We talked to the country's top trainers and asked them to help us design a workout plan devoted entirely to better sex.

It's true that *any* weight lifting plan will go a long way toward boosting the endurance and strength that you need for good sex, but most of the exercise you get in the bedroom brings specific muscle groups into play. When you tone and strengthen these muscles, you'll find that you'll be able to have sex longer than you did before. You'll have more energy. You'll be able to hold yourself in the most common sexual positions without fatigue.

This program is simple, yet it hits every major muscle group. It's divided into two phases. Phase 1 concentrates on building your strength base. Even if you do nothing else, it will give you strength and flexibility in places you never had them—and you (and your partner) will notice the difference within a few weeks, in bed and out.

Once you've mastered the exercises in Phase 1—for most men, it will take several months, although some of you might be ready after 4 to 6 weeks—it's time to concentrate on specific muscles. Narrowing your focus to specific muscles will tone and sculpt your body, while at the same time improving your strength and endurance when the lights go down.

What about the "Position of Strength" exercises you see at the end of this chapter? How do those fit into the plan? The most effective way to incorporate those into your workouts is to prioritize them by starting each workout with one or two of the exercises.

As you'll see in the charts after each workout, this program requires working out 4 days a week. We've divided the charts into "Day One" and "Day Two" workouts, each of which will be repeated twice a week, giving you time off in between.

As for equipment, you'll need either access to a gym or a nicely appointed home setup. If you don't have either, do the at-home variations. All you'll need are some water bottles; soup cans; and heavy boxes, suitcases, sandbags, or cinder blocks. Or you might consider buying a set of dumbbells and some resistance bands. All told, they won't cost nearly as much as a home gym or gym membership.

PHASE 1

# LOWER BODY ▶

**THIS IS THE PLACE TO START FOR BETTER SEX.** The most powerful muscles in your body are in the lower body. It makes sense because just about every position you find yourself in, sexual or otherwise, puts at least some strain on the legs, hips, and butt. These are also the muscles that give the power and strength to maintain and change sexual positions.

### PHASE 1: LOWER BODY

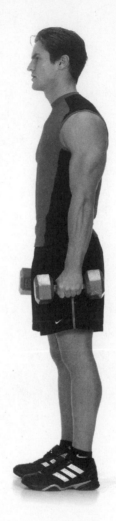

## DUMBBELL LUNGE

**START:** Grab a dumbbell in each hand, with your palms facing your body, and stand with your feet hip-width apart.

**FINISH:** Keeping your back straight, take a long step forward with your right leg. Bend your leg until your right thigh is parallel with the floor. Your left leg should be extended, with your knee slightly bent and almost touching the floor. Keep your right foot stationary as you straighten your right leg. Switch legs and repeat on the other side.

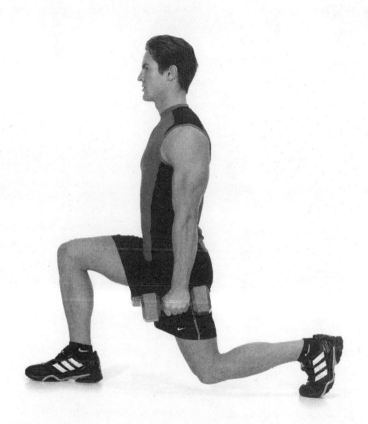

**AT-HOME VARIATION:** Substitute full plastic water or detergent bottles or unopened soup cans, depending on how heavy you want the weight to be. (Not pictured.)

▶*Sexual Gains:* **This exercise works the butt and the front of the thigh, while putting little stress on the knee. It also strengthens the hamstrings, improves balance and posture, and supports missionary, standing, and kneeling positions.**

## PHASE 1: LOWER BODY

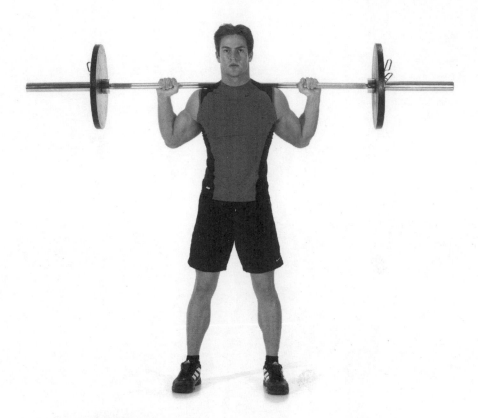

## BARBELL SQUAT

**START:** Place a barbell at shoulder level on a squat rack. Grip the bar with your hands slightly more than shoulder-width apart, palms facing front. Step under the bar so that it's evenly positioned across your upper back and shoulders, not your neck. Stand up straight with your feet hip-width apart and your knees slightly bent. Don't drop your head; keep it in line with your torso.

**FINISH:** Keeping your feet flat and torso straight, bend your knees slightly and squat down as though sitting in a chair behind you. Don't allow your knees to extend past your toes. Continue moving downward until your thighs are parallel with the floor. Then slowly rise to a standing position.

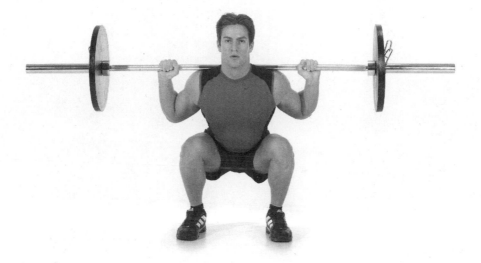

**AT-HOME VARIATION:** Wall Squat (page 164)

▶*Sexual Gains:* **All told, the squat works more than 200 different muscles. It is the main exercise used by elite athletes for strengthening the large muscle groups—specifically, the front thigh (quadriceps), butt, and hamstrings. It also works the calves and shins, along with muscles in the shoulders, arms, and back. Great for standing and athletic positions.**

## PHASE 1: LOWER BODY

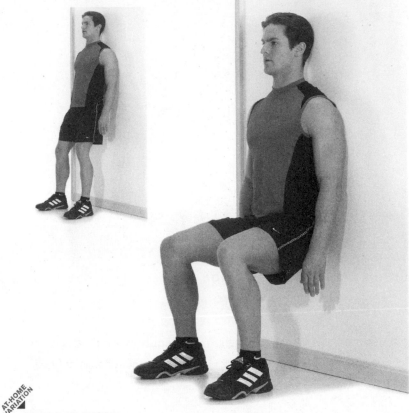

AT-HOME VARIATION ►

## WALL SQUAT

**START:** Stand with your back flat against a wall, with your feet a little wider than shoulder-width apart and your toes pointed slightly outward. Bend at your knees, keeping your weight centered over your feet.

**FINISH:** Lower your body as resistance, until your knees are bent 90 degrees. Straighten up slowly, concentrating on using your legs to slide up the wall. *Note:* Holding a heavy object—a couple of filled water bottles, for example—will give you more resistance.

PHASE 1

# UPPER BODY ▶

**JUST AS YOU CAN'T HAVE GOOD SEX WITHOUT A STRONG LOWER BODY, YOU CAN'T HOPE TO PERFORM AT YOUR BEST UNLESS YOUR BACK, CHEST, AND ARMS ARE EQUALLY STRONG.** It's especially important to work the back, an area men tend to neglect. When properly strengthened and defined, the muscles give the back a visually pleasing V shape, which has the added benefit of making your waist look smaller.

## PHASE 1: UPPER BODY

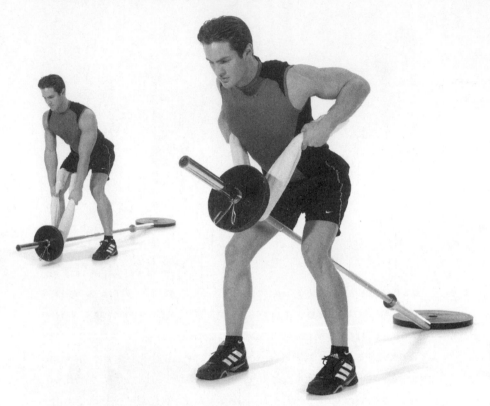

## BENT-OVER ROW

**START:** Using an Olympic-size (45-pound) bar, wedge one end in a corner and place a 25-pound or lighter weight plate on the other end. Wrap a towel around the bar, just under the weight plate. Straddle the bar, keeping your knees slightly bent. Your chin should be up, your chest out, stomach in, shoulders back, and back flat.

**FINISH:** Pull the bar to your chest, slightly arching your back and letting your elbows rise above your chest. Slowly lower the bar to arm's length, then repeat.

**AT-HOME VARIATION:** Suitcase Row (opposite)

▶*Sexual Gains:* **Improves posture and form and is particularly important for vigorous sex, which tends to put a lot of pressure on the lower back.**

PHASE **1**: UPPER BODY

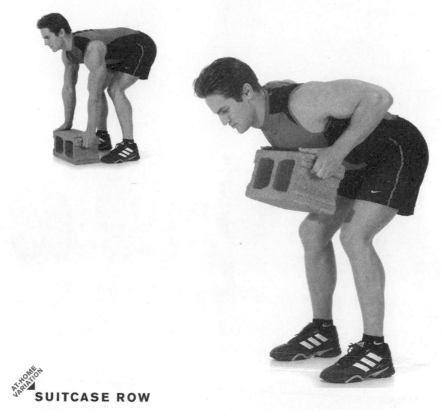

**SUITCASE ROW**

**START:** Set a full suitcase (or sandbag, cinder block, railroad tie, whatever) in front of you. Stand with your legs comfortably apart, then bend over at your hips, with your knees bent and your back flat, and grab the sides of the bag.

**FINISH:** Use your back and biceps to pull the suitcase up to your chest, keeping it close to your body. Pause, then slowly return to the starting position.

PHASE **1**: UPPER BODY

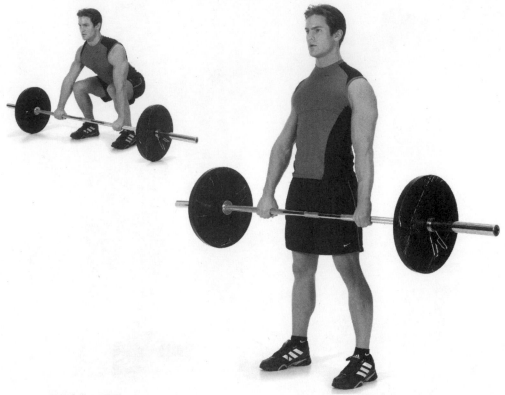

## DEADLIFT

**START:** Load a barbell and set it on the floor. Squat behind it with your feet shoulder-width apart. Grab it overhand, with your hands just outside your legs, your shoulders over or just behind the bar, your arms straight, and your back flat or slightly arched.

**FINISH:** Straighten up, lifting the weight to a standing position. Push with your heels and pull the weight to your body as you stand. Pause, then slowly return to the starting position.

**AT-HOME VARIATION:** Boxlift (opposite)

▶*Sexual Gains:* **This is another superb exercise for strengthening all of the major back muscles, important for energetic sex. Be sure to do this exercise slowly. You defeat its purpose if you use momentum to finish your reps.**

PHASE 1: UPPER BODY

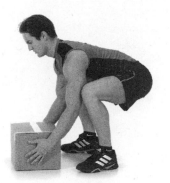

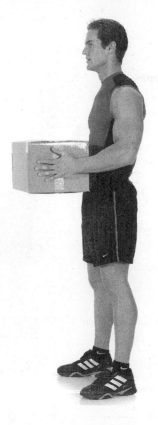

 AT-HOME VARIATION

## BOXLIFT

**START:** Set a weighted box on the floor. Stand behind the box, with your feet shoulder-width apart and your toes pointed out slightly. Squat behind the box and grab it with a neutral grip (palms facing each other).

**FINISH:** Straighten up, lifting the box to a standing position. Push with your heels and pull the weight to your body as you stand. Pause, then slowly return to the starting position.

PHASE 1: UPPER BODY

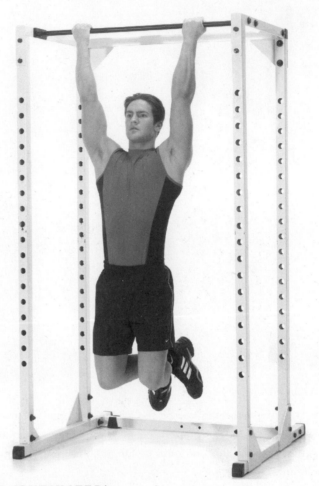

## CHINUP (SUPINATED)

**START:** Using an underhand grip, grab a chinup bar and place your hands shoulder-width apart. Hang from the bar with your elbows slightly bent and your ankles crossed.

**FINISH:** Slowly pull yourself up until your chin is over the bar. Hold for a second or two, then slowly return to the starting position.

**AT-HOME VARIATION:** At-home variations for Chinups are not really practical. You're much better off purchasing a chinup bar.

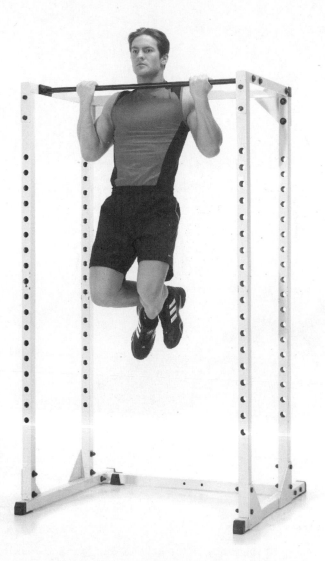

▶*Sexual Gains:* Chinups look easy, but they require you to raise your entire body weight. They work all of the major upper- and mid-body muscles, including those in the back, chest, and arms. You need a strong back and chest to support yourself in the man-on-top position. Your partner will get a visual treat because most women are attracted to a well-developed chest.

## PHASE 1: UPPER BODY

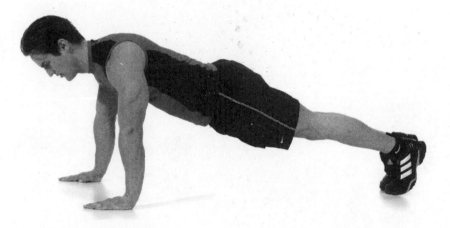

## PUSHUP

**START:** Support your body on the balls of your feet and your hands, positioning the latter slightly wider than shoulder-width apart, palms flat on the floor. Keep your eyes on the floor and your legs, back, and neck in a straight line.

**FINISH:** Lower your torso until your chest almost touches the floor, then slowly return to the starting position.

**TO WORK YOUR CHEST MORE:** Place your hands more than shoulder-width apart.

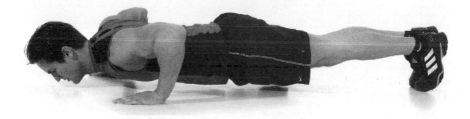

**TO WORK YOUR BACK AND ARMS MORE:** Place your hands together underneath your chest, thumbs and index fingers touching.

**AT-HOME VARIATION:** Not necessary. You can do Pushups anywhere, anytime.

▶*Sexual Gains:* **Besides supporting you in the man-on-top position and all its variations, a strong chest and arms are required for standing positions in which you lift your partner off the floor.**

## PHASE 1: UPPER BODY

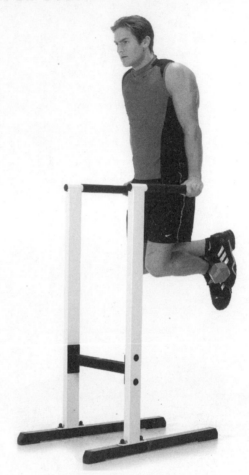

## DIP

**START:** Using the parallel bars or dip station at the gym, grab the handles with a neutral grip. Jump up and steady yourself. Start the movement with your arms straight but not locked and your body perfectly still. You can cross your legs behind you or leave them hanging straight down. The more upright you are, the harder you work your triceps. Leaning forward shifts the work to your chest and shoulders.

**FINISH:** Slowly lower your body until your upper arms are parallel with the floor. Push back up to the starting position. You can make

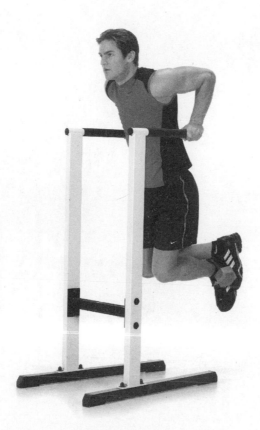

the move harder by wearing a weighted dip belt or clenching a dumbbell between your ankles.

**AT-HOME VARIATION:** Table Dip (page 176)

▶*Sexual Gains:* **Dips build a strong chest, arms, and shoulders. Specifically, they work the deltoid muscles in your shoulders. They're the key to moving your arms, and they play a central role in many sexual positions, including man on top. Surprisingly, your shoulder muscles come into play when you're performing oral sex if you're propped up on your elbows.**

## PHASE 1: UPPER BODY

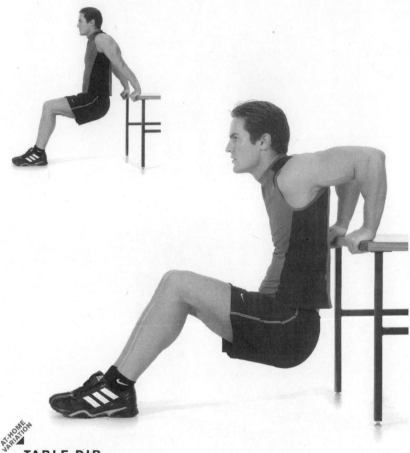

AT-HOME VARIATION

### TABLE DIP

**START:** Position your hands shoulder-width apart on a secure table, palms down. Walk your feet out so that your knees form a 90-degree angle.

**FINISH:** Lower your torso until your butt is within an inch of the floor. Slowly return to the starting position.

## PHASE 1: UPPER BODY

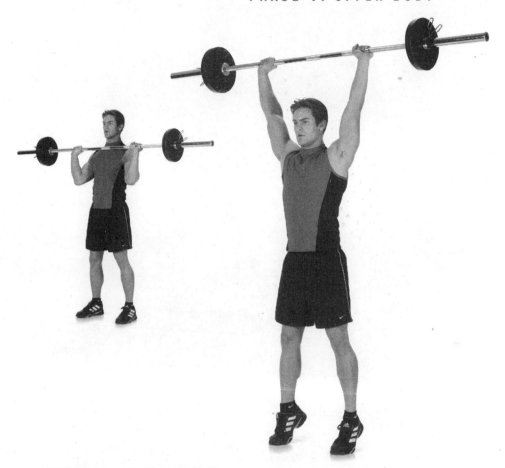

## BARBELL PUSH PRESS

**START:** Balance a barbell on the fronts of your shoulders, with your hands shoulder-width apart and your elbows pointed up. Your knees should be slightly bent.

**FINISH:** Push the bar straight up until your elbows are almost locked. At the same time, rise slightly on your toes. Then slowly return to the starting position.

**AT-HOME VARIATION:** Anterior Pushup (page 178)

▶*Sexual Gains:* **Another great exercise for increasing the shoulder strength you need for man-on-top positions.**

## PHASE 1: UPPER BODY

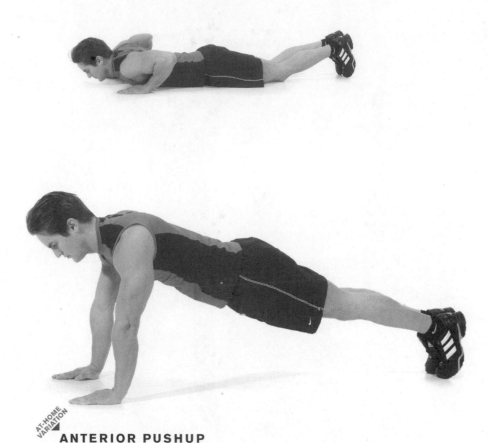

AT-HOME VARIATION

## ANTERIOR PUSHUP

**START:** Lie facedown on the floor, with your hands flat under your shoulders and your toes touching the floor.

**FINISH:** Push off the floor by extending your arms, keeping your body and legs stiff. Use only your palms and toes to hold your body up. While in the arms-extended position, round your back (this will add another inch off the floor). Finally, retract your shoulder blades, then bend your arms slowly, lowering your chest until it just barely touches the floor. Push back up again and repeat.

▶*Sexual Gains:* **A variation of the Barbell Push Press, this is another great exercise for increasing shoulder strength.**

## ABDOMINALS ▶

**THE ABDOMINAL MUSCLES ARE WHAT ALLOW YOU TO BEND FORWARD, BACKWARD, AND SIDE TO SIDE.** Sexually, they're the muscles that provide strong thrusting power, while at the same time allowing you to subtly alter your position and angle of thrust.

Of course, to take best advantage of your abs, you should first lose your gut. *"My sex life is better now that my gut isn't in the way for either of us,"* says a 58-year-old retired high school principal who embarked on a weight-loss plan along with an ab-strengthening workout.

Once the gut starts to go, you'll notice that there is quite a number of muscles hidden away in there. The major ones include the transversus abdominis, which helps keep the abdominal wall tight and allows you to maintain a firm erection and control premature ejaculation. The quadratis lumborum are muscles that allow you to bend to each side. The rectus abdominis, or six-pack muscle, is the large, flat muscle running the length of the abdomen that promotes trunk flexion. The external abdominal obliques are muscles that run down the sides and front of the abdomen and allow your body to rotate and bend from side to side. The internal abdominal obliques also enable sideways movements.

Working on all these muscles has clear sexual benefits. *"I've definitely noticed increased endurance, ability, and range of motion through increases in core strength,"* a 29-year-old computer programmer told us.

## PHASE 1: ABDOMINALS

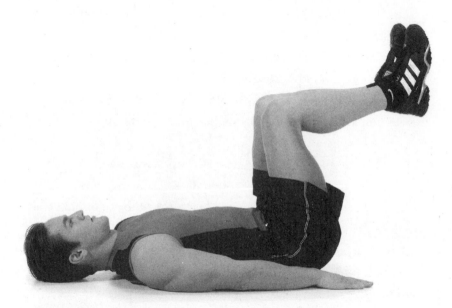

## REVERSE CRUNCH

**START:** Lie on your back, with your arms by your sides. Hold your legs off the floor with your knees bent at a 90-degree angle so your thighs point straight up and your lower legs point straight ahead, parallel with the floor.

**FINISH:** Roll your pelvis backward and raise your hips a few inches off the floor; your knees should be over your chest. Hold for a moment, then return to the starting position.

**AT-HOME VARIATION:** Not necessary. You can do most ab exercises anywhere, anytime.

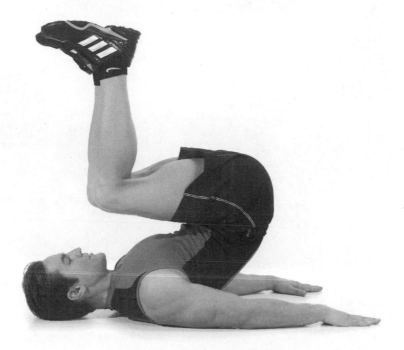

▶*Sexual Gains:* This is among the best exercises for strengthening the lower abdominals, and it's among the easiest. It improves your thrusting endurance and fine-tunes subtle thrusting movements.

PHASE **1**: ABDOMINALS

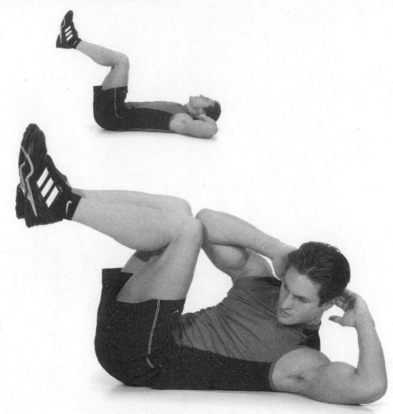

## TWISTING OBLIQUE CRUNCH

**START:** Lie on your back, with your hands loosely touching the back of your head or neck. Bend your knees at a 90-degree angle.

**FINISH:** Lift your upper body off the floor and twist to the left, until your right elbow touches your left knee. Slowly return to the starting position, then repeat in the opposite direction.

**AT-HOME VARIATION:** Not necessary.

▶*Sexual Gains:* **This exercise strengthens your obliques and is good for side-by-side positions in which you enter your partner from behind and reach around her to stimulate her clitoris. You also use your obliques anytime you attempt some of the more acrobatic positions.**

PHASE 1: ABDOMINALS

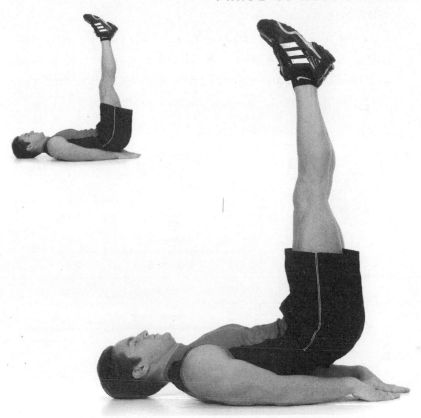

## PULSE-UP

**START:** Lie with your hands flat underneath your tailbone and your legs pointed straight up toward the ceiling, perpendicular to your torso.

**FINISH:** Pull your navel inward and flex your glutes as you lift your hips just a few inches off the floor. Then lower your hips.

**AT-HOME VARIATION:** Not necessary.

▶*Sexual Gains:* **Good for thrusting endurance and subtle thrusting movements.**

## PHASE 1
## WORKOUT PLAN

It's a good idea to warm up before launching into any strength-training workout. Walk briskly, or ride an exercise bike for at least 5 to 10 minutes. It's also a good idea to stretch when the workout is done. See chapter 5 for a complete guide to stretching.

## DAY ONE

| EXERCISE | SETS | REPS | REP SPEED (SECONDS) | REST INTERVAL |
|---|---|---|---|---|
| Chinup (supinated) | 2 | 10–12 | 2 down, 3 up | 1 min. |
| Barbell Squat | 2 | 10–12 | 2 down, 3 up | 1 min. |
| Pushup | 2 | 10–12 | 2 down, 3 up | 1 min. |
| Deadlift | 2 | 10–12 | 2 down, 3 up | 2 min. |
| Pulse-Up | 2 | 10–12 | hold 3 at top | 10 sec. |
| Reverse Crunch | 2 | 10–12 | 2 down, 3 up | 1½ min. |

## DAY TWO

| EXERCISE | SETS | REPS | REP SPEED (SECONDS) | REST INTERVAL |
|---|---|---|---|---|
| Barbell Push Press | 2 | 10–12 | 3 down, explode up | 1 min. |
| Dumbbell Lunge | 2 | 10–12 | 2 down, explode up | 1 min. |
| Dip | 2 | 10–12 | 2 down, 3 up | 1 min. |
| Bent-Over Row | 2 | 10–12 | 2 down, 3 up | 2 min. |
| Twisting Oblique Crunch | 2 | 10–12 | 2 down, 2 up | 1 min. |

PHASE **2**

## LOWER BODY ▶

**ONCE YOU'VE MASTERED THE EXERCISES IN PHASE 1, WHICH FOR MOST MEN WILL TAKE SEVERAL MONTHS, MOVE ON TO PHASE 2.** Here's where you'll start concentrating on specific muscles. As in phase 1, phase 2 has lower body, upper body, and abdominals sections, along with a biceps and triceps section.

## PHASE 2: LOWER BODY

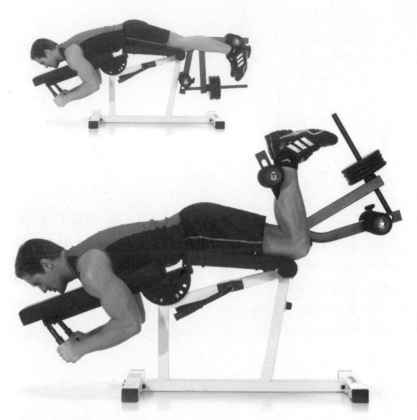

## LEG CURL

**START:** Lie facedown on a leg-curl machine.

**FINISH:** With your hips flat against the bench and your abdominal muscles tight, curl your legs behind you until your feet are about perpendicular to the bench. Pause, then lower your legs slowly to the starting position, stopping just before your knees are straight.

**AT-HOME VARIATION:** Dumbbell Leg Curl (opposite)

▶ *Sexual Gains:* **Strong hamstrings are essential for standing and kneeling positions.**

PHASE **2**: LOWER BODY

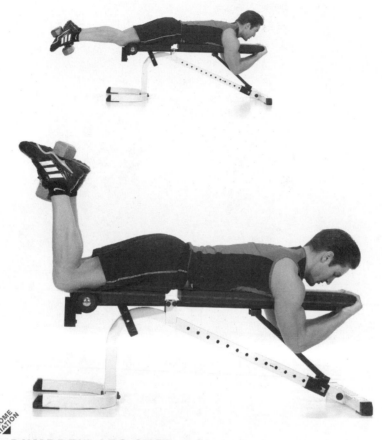

AT-HOME VARIATION

## DUMBBELL LEG CURL

**START:** Set a dumbbell between the insteps of your feet and lie facedown on a flat bench. (This is tricky at first, and you might need someone to help you.) Grab the front or sides of the bench for support.

**FINISH:** Keeping your hips against the bench, curl the weight up toward your butt. Stop when your lower legs point straight up, then, without pausing, lower the weight slowly.

PHASE **2**: LOWER BODY

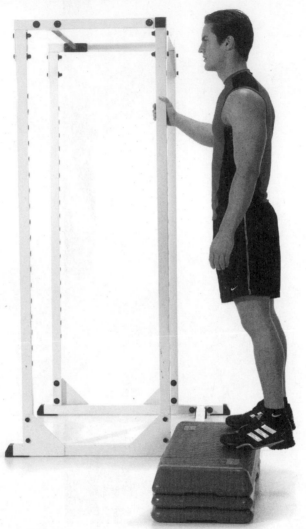

## CALF RAISE

**START:** Stand with the balls of your feet on the edge of a step, with your legs about 12 inches apart. Hold onto the banister or wall for stability.

**FINISH:** Slowly rise on your toes as far as you can go, hold for a second, then lower yourself back. To work different portions of the calves, shift your feet so that your toes point either in or out.

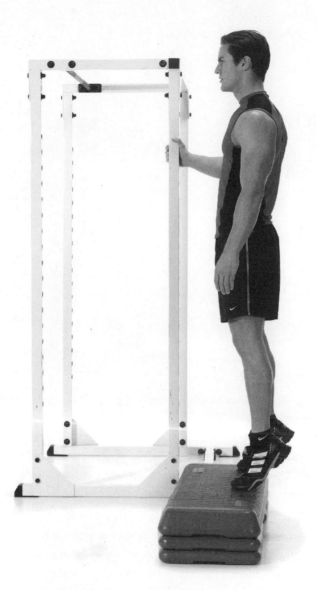

**AT-HOME VARIATION:** Not necessary.

▶*Sexual Gains:* **Strong calves improve your endurance and strength for standing positions.**

PHASE **2**: UPPER BODY

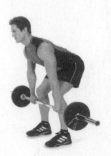

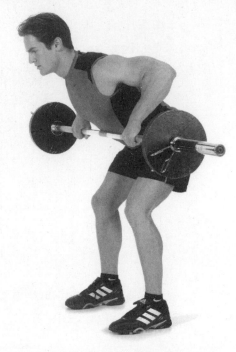

## BENT-OVER ROW

**START:** Stand with your feet shoulder-width apart and your knees bent 15 to 30 degrees. Keep your torso straight, with a slight arch in your back, as you lean forward at the hips. Try to get your torso close to parallel with the floor. Grab the barbell off the floor with a full overhand grip (thumbs wrapped around the bar) that's slightly wider than shoulder width. Let the bar hang at arm's length in front of you.

**FINISH:** Retract your shoulder blades to start pulling the bar up to the lower part of your sternum (breastbone). Pause at the top, with your chest sticking out toward the bar. Slowly return to the starting position. Try to keep your torso in the same position throughout the movement.

**AT-HOME VARIATION:** Suitcase Row (opposite)

▶*Sexual Gains:* **Good for strengthening and sculpting the lower and middle portions of the back. Again, a strong back is essential for standing or kneeling positions and important for stamina during any vigorous lovemaking session.**

PHASE **2**: UPPER BODY

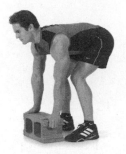

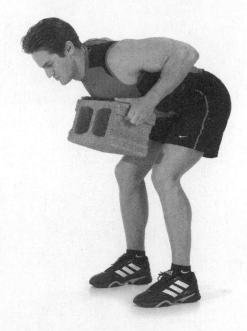

AT-HOME VARIATION

## SUITCASE ROW

**START:** Set a full suitcase (or sandbag, cinder block, railroad tie, whatever) in front of you. Stand with your legs comfortably apart, then bend over at your hips, with your knees bent and your back flat, and grab the sides of the bag.

**FINISH:** Use your back and biceps to pull the suitcase up to your chest, keeping it close to your body. Pause, then slowly return to the starting position.

PHASE **2**: UPPER BODY

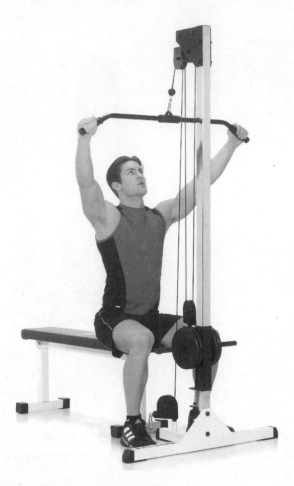

## LATERAL PULLDOWN

**START:** Sit at a lat pulldown machine. Grasp the bar with your hands about shoulder-width apart and a false overhand grip (thumbs on the same side of the bar as your fingers). Your arms should be fully extended overhead and your torso upright or leaning back slightly.

**FINISH:** Pull the bar straight down until it almost touches your upper chest, while squeezing your shoulder blades together. Slowly return to the starting position with your chest out, keeping full control of the bar at all times.

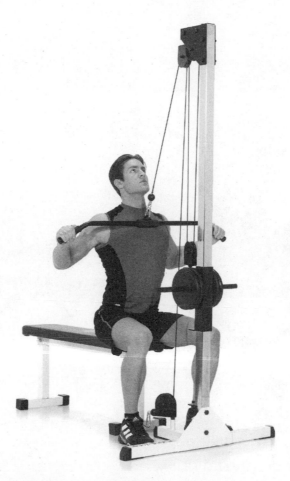

**AT-HOME VARIATION:** Dumbbell Pullover (page 194)

▶*Sexual Gains:* This exercise works the upper part of the back, along with the shoulders and arms. It's another great exercise for man-on-top positions and standing positions in which you lift your partner off the floor.

PHASE **2**: UPPER BODY

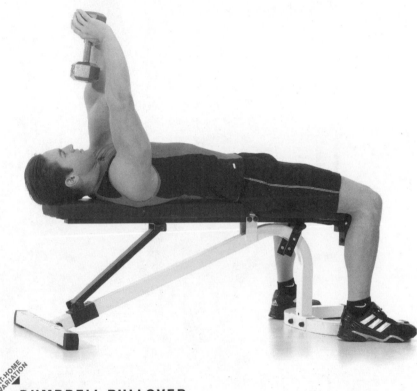

AT-HOME VARIATION

## DUMBBELL PULLOVER

**START:** Lie flat on a bench. Press your head, torso, lower back, and glutes firmly against the surface. Your feet should be flat on the floor (or, if you prefer, the end of the bench). Place one hand around the handle of a dumbbell, then wrap the other over the gripping hand. Extend your arms directly above your collarbone, holding the dumbbell perpendicular to the floor.

**FINISH:** Keeping your back flat against the bench to elongate your lats, slowly lower the weight behind your head until your arms are in

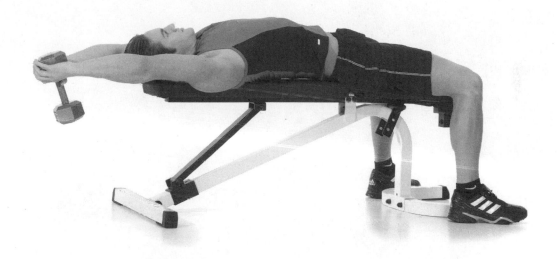

line with your ears. Pause, then pull the weight back up. Slightly bend your elbows throughout.

▶*Sexual Gains:* **This exercise is a variation of the Lateral Pulldown that can be done at home. It works the upper part of the back, along with the shoulders and arms.**

## PHASE 2: UPPER BODY

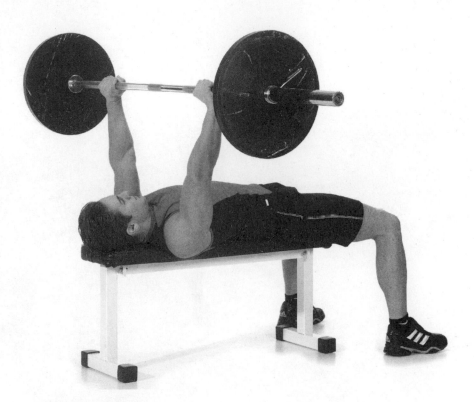

## BENCH PRESS

**START:** Lie flat on a bench, with your feet flat on the floor and your head positioned about eye level under the bar. Grab the barbell with a full overhand grip (thumbs wrapped around the bar), placing your hands about shoulder-width apart. Remove the bar from the uprights and hold it with straight arms over your collarbone. Pull your shoulder blades together in back.

**FINISH:** Lower the bar, slowly and in control, to just above your nipples. Then press it up and slightly back so it finishes above your

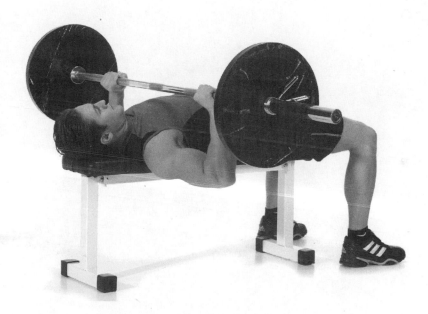

collarbone again. Stop just short of locking your elbows, and keep
your shoulder blades pulled back.

**AT-HOME VARIATION:** Use dumbbells, filled water bottles,
or unopened soup cans. (Not pictured.)

▶*Sexual Gains:* **The Bench Press is the main exercise for
building a bigger chest, which not only looks great when you're
on top but also helps hold you up.**

## PHASE 2: UPPER BODY

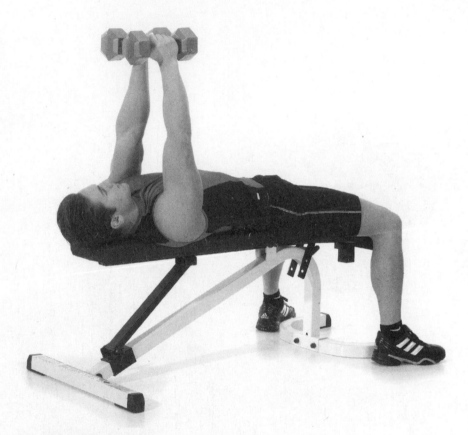

### DUMBBELL FLY

**START:** Grab a pair of dumbbells that are lighter than those you'd use for a dumbbell bench press. Lie flat on a bench, with your feet flat on the floor and the dumbbells at arm's length above your chest.

**FINISH:** Maintaining a slight bend in your elbows, lower the dumbbells down and back until your upper arms are parallel with the floor and in line with your ears. Pause for a moment, then use your chest to pull the weights back to the starting position, repeating your movements in reverse. Keep your shoulder blades

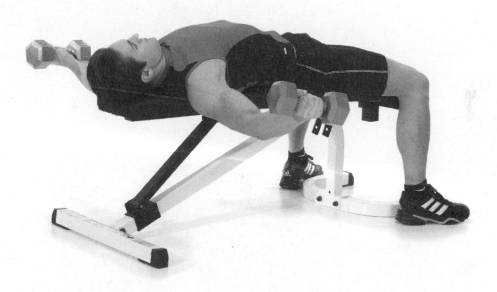

pulled toward each other throughout, and flex your pecs at the top of the movement.

**AT-HOME VARIATION:** Substitute unopened soup cans or filled water bottles for the dumbbells. (Not pictured.)

▶*Sexual Gains:* **This is similar to the Bench Press, except you have to balance the dumbbells separately—which works your chest muscles even more.**

PHASE **2**: UPPER BODY

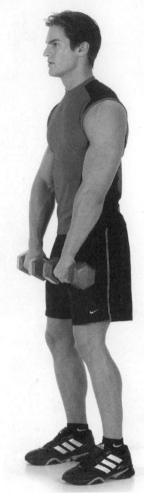

## DUMBBELL FRONT RAISE

**START:** Grab a dumbbell in each hand, with your arms hanging in front of your thighs. Stand with your feet shoulder-width apart, knees slightly bent, and lean forward very slightly at the hips (to avoid leaning back as you lift).

**FINISH:** Bend your elbows slightly and raise the dumbbells straight in front of you until your arms are parallel with the floor. Pause, then slowly return to the starting position.

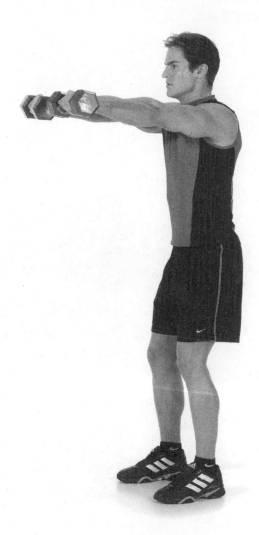

**AT-HOME VARIATION:** Substitute unopened soup cans or filled water bottles for the dumbbells. (Not pictured.)

▶ *Sexual Gains:* **This exercise puts power and definition in your shoulders—and you get an extra workout because you have to balance the dumbbells separately. It's especially good for when you're in the man-on-top position for an extended period of time.**

PHASE 2: UPPER BODY

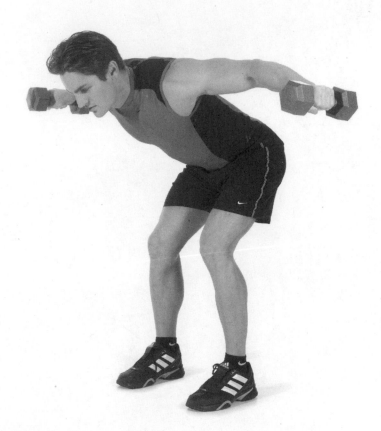

## BENT-OVER LATERAL RAISE

**START:** Sit or stand, with your torso bent forward almost parallel with the floor and your knees slightly spread. Grab a dumbbell in each hand with your palms facing inward, elbows slightly bent.

**FINISH:** Slowly raise the dumbbells out to your sides, keeping your elbows bent, your back straight, and your head in a neutral position. Squeeze your shoulder blades together at the highest point in the movement. Pause, then slowly lower the dumbbells to the starting position.

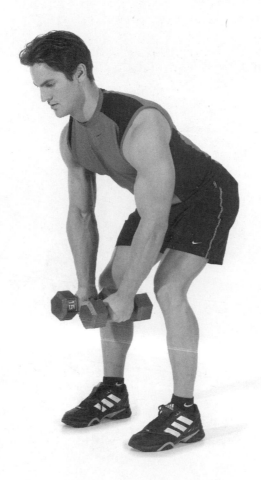

**AT-HOME VARIATION:** Substitute unopened soup cans or filled water bottles for the dumbbells. (Not pictured.)

▶*Sexual Gains:* **This exercise hits the shoulders at a slightly different angle than the Front Raise, giving you that much extra man-on-top staying power. This exercise is also good for strengthening the muscles that support your neck when you're performing oral sex.**

## PHASE 2: BICEPS AND TRICEPS

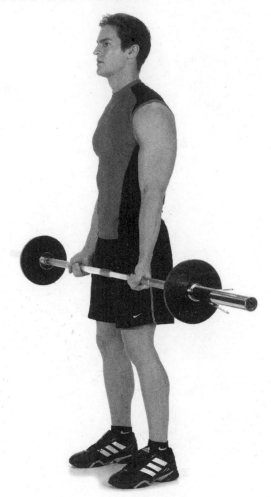

## BICEPS CURL

**START:** Holding a barbell or dumbbells with an underhand grip, stand with your feet shoulder-width apart and your arms down at your sides.

**FINISH:** Curl your arms up toward your shoulders. Stop and squeeze when the weight is 6 to 8 inches from your shoulders. Keep your abdomen tight, your elbows still, and your upper body straight. Pause, then lower the weight to the starting position.

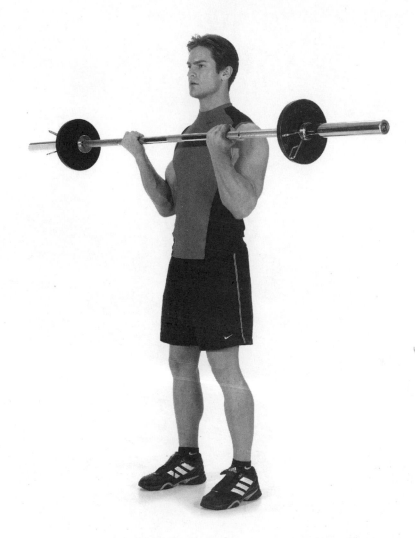

**AT-HOME VARIATION:** Substitute unopened soup cans or filled water bottles for the barbell or dumbbells. (Not pictured.)

▶*Sexual Gains:* **Strong biceps are necessary for lifting your partner, man-on-top positions, and rear-entry positions in which you support yourself with your arms.**

## PHASE 2: BICEPS AND TRICEPS

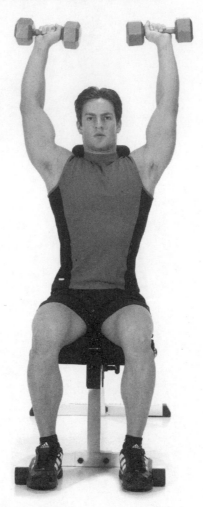

## SEATED DUMBBELL TRICEPS EXTENSION

**START:** Sit on a bench with a 90-degree back support. With a neutral, shoulder-width grip, grab a pair of dumbbells and hold them straight up over your head with your elbows unlocked.

**FINISH:** Bend at the elbows as you lower the weights down to the sides of your head. Keep your upper arms in the same position and pause when your elbows are bent just past 90 degrees. Return to the starting position.

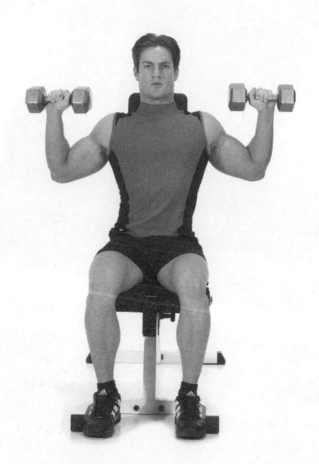

**AT-HOME VARIATION:** Use filled water bottles or unopened soup cans. (Not pictured.)

▶*Sexual Gains:* **Triceps are harder to build than biceps, but you need balanced strength in your arms for maximum muscle power for lifting your partner, man-on-top, and rear-entry positions.**

## PHASE 2: BICEPS AND TRICEPS

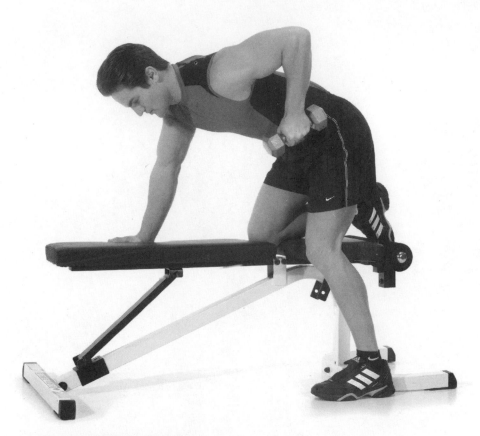

## TRICEPS KICKBACK

**START:** Grab a light dumbbell in your left hand and place your right hand and knee on a bench. Plant your left foot on the floor. Bend forward at the hips so your torso is parallel with the floor. Hold the dumbbell at your side with a neutral grip, elbow pointed toward the ceiling.

**FINISH:** Lift the weight up and back until your arm is straight. Keep your elbow pointed toward the ceiling and the rest of your body steady. Pause for 2 full seconds, then slowly return to the starting position. Finish the set on the left side before repeating on the right.

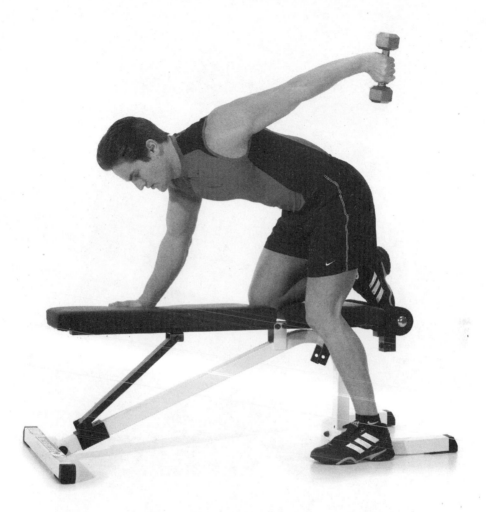

**AT-HOME VARIATION:** Substitute unopened soup cans or filled water bottles for the dumbbells. (Not pictured.)

▶*Sexual Gains:* **Besides needing strong arms to lift your partner or support yourself when you're on top, you also need them during foreplay. You can stimulate your partner manually for much longer if your arms don't get tired.**

## PHASE 2: ABDOMINALS

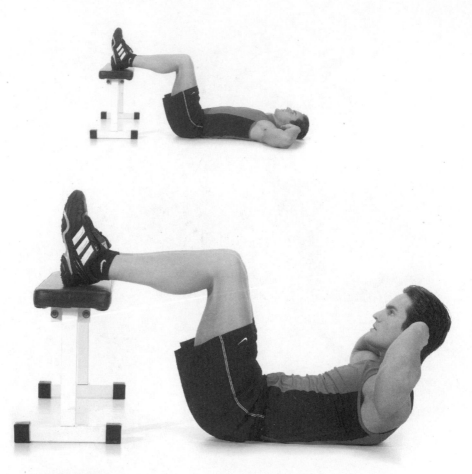

## CRUNCH

**START:** Lie on your back, with your knees bent at 90 degrees or resting on a bench. Hold your hands behind your ears.

**FINISH:** Use your abs to curl your torso upward 4 to 6 inches, keeping your lower back firmly pressed to the floor. Pause, then slowly lower your back to the floor.

**AT-HOME VARIATION:** Not necessary.

▶*Sexual Gains:* **This is the core exercise for building strong abs. Two words: Thrusting power.**

PHASE 2: ABDOMINALS

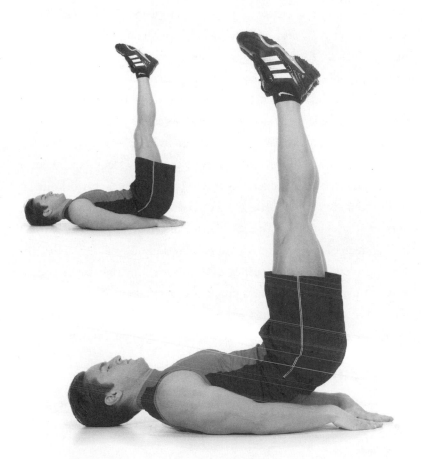

## PULSE-UP

**START:** Lie with your hands underneath your tailbone and your legs pointed straight up toward the ceiling, perpendicular to your torso.

**FINISH:** Pull your navel inward and flex your glutes as you lift your hips just a few inches off the floor. Then lower your hips.

**AT-HOME VARIATION:** Not necessary.

▶*Sexual Gains:* **Good for thrusting endurance and subtle thrusting movements.**

## PHASE 2
## WORKOUT PLAN

Because this phase of the sexual fitness plan is more vigorous than the first, don't rush into it. Work your way through Phase 1 until your muscles no longer feel sore from lactic acid buildup after a workout, roughly 4 to 6 weeks after you start Phase 1.

Phase 2 is divided into push and pull days. On push days, work your chest, shoulders, and triceps—with exercises in which you push the weight. On pull days, work your back and biceps—with exercises that pull weight. Do the lower-body exercises on the second day. Plan on doing the abdominal exercises toward the end of each workout.

Don't be afraid to shuffle the exercises. Varying your workout every few weeks will hit muscles from different angles and with varying degrees of intensity, providing new stimuli ideal for optimal muscle growth. If you're satisfied with the strength and size of your arms, for example, substitute a couple of extra leg or abdominal exercises. Or maybe you're just not getting the results you need from the reverse crunch. Replace it with regular abdominal crunches.

## DAY ONE (PUSH)

| EXERCISE | SETS | REPS | REP SPEED (SECONDS) | REST INTERVAL |
|---|---|---|---|---|
| Bench Press | 2 | 10–12 | 2 down, 3 up | 1 min. |
| Bent-Over Lateral Raise | 2 | 10–12 | 2 down, 3 up | 1 min. |
| Dip | 2 | 10–12 | 2 down, 3 up | 1 min. |
| Seated Dumbbell Triceps Ext. | 2 | 10–12 | 2 down, 3 up | 1 min. |
| Dumbbell Front Raise | 2 | 10–12 | 2 down, 3 up | 1 min. |
| Triceps Kickback | 2 | 10–12 | 2 down, 3 up | 1 min. |
| Crunch | 2 | 10–12 | hold 3 at top | 10 sec. |
| Pulse-Up | 2 | 10–12 | hold 3 at top | 10 sec. |
| Dumbell Fly | 2 | 10–12 | 2 down, 3 up | 1 min. |

## DAY TWO (PULL)

| EXERCISE | SETS | REPS | REP SPEED (SEC) | REST INTERVAL |
|---|---|---|---|---|
| Barbell Squat | 2 | 10–12 | 2 down, explode up | 1 min. |
| Leg Curl | 2 | 10–12 | 2 down, 3 up | 1 min. |
| Biceps Curl | 2 | 10–12 | 2 down, 3 up | 1 min. |
| Bent-Over Row 2 | 2 | 10–12 | 2 down, 3 up | 2 min. |
| Lateral Pulldown | 2 | 10–12 | 2 down, 3 up | 1 min. |
| Calf Raise | 2 | 10–12 | 2 down, 3 up | 1 min. |
| Reverse Crunch | 2 | 10–12 | 2 down, 2 up | 1 min. |
| Twisting Oblique Crunch | 2 | 10–12 | 2 down, 2 up | 1 min. |

# POSITIONS OF STRENGTH ▶

After a dizzying 54 pages of workouts, how can there be more? The next 13 exercises are specifically targeted to sexual positions mentioned in this book and are the most effective workout for the position they're paired with. For example, the missionary position works best if you support your weight over your partner's body, leaving some space in between. What bears the bulk of that effort? Your shoulders—and the best exercise to strengthen them is the lateral raise.

The positions we chose range from everyday basic to spice-it-up complex. We picked perennial favorites (missionary, woman on top) as well as ones we think you'll like even if you don't try them more than once (the Honeybee, the Pretzel).

You can incorporate each exercise into the workouts described earlier in this chapter by prioritizing one or two each day at the beginning of your workout. Or, if you're not up for the full exercise program for whatever reason, pick the exercise that supports your favorite position and do that one only. That's an ideal strategy for when you don't have a lot of time to work out or you're on the road or under the weather. Even if you can't get a full workout in, your sex life won't suffer.

# *Man on Top* *(page 2)*

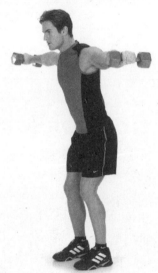

*Why she likes it: Deep penetration, ease of kissing, body-to-body closeness. The so-called missionary position hardly indicates a lack of creativity. Surveys show it's a perennial favorite of men as well as women. In this position, you also can press your pubic bone against her clitoris as you rock and thrust, giving her extreme pleasure.*

**MUSCLES TO WORK:** Shoulders. They keep your torso upright and keep your full weight off her body. Also, your naked chest and abs give her extra visual pleasure.

**BEST WORKOUT:** Standing Lateral Raises. Stand holding a pair of dumbbells at your sides with an overhand grip, your elbows slightly bent. Bend slightly forward at the hips, keeping your lower back in its naturally arched position. Raise your arms up and out to the sides until they're parallel with the floor, keeping the same bend in your elbows. Pause, then slowly return to the starting position. Try for three sets of eight repetitions each.

# *Woman on Top* (page 8)

*Why she likes it:* She controls the pace and movements.

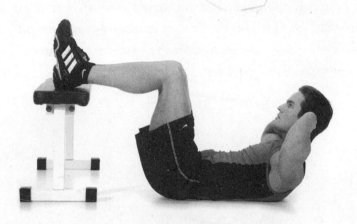

**MUSCLES TO WORK:** Abdominals. They provide good thrusting control and force—important when you're in the passive position, without the leverage you have on top.

**BEST WORKOUT:** Crunches. Lie on your back, with your knees bent at 90 degrees or resting on a bench. Hold your hands behind your ears. Use your abs to curl your torso upward 4 to 6 inches, keeping your lower back firmly pressed to the floor. Pause, then slowly lower. Try to start with three sets of 10 crunches. As your endurance increases, increase it to five sets of 20.

# *Woman on Top, Back to Front* (page 12)

*Why she likes it: There's deep penetration, she controls the pace, and she can stimulate her clitoris manually. In this classic Eastern position, you lie on your back as the woman straddles your penis, her bottom toward your face.*

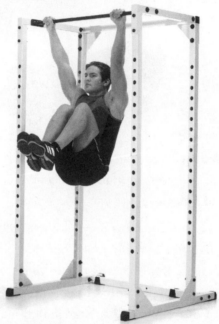

**MUSCLES TO WORK:** Hips, abdominals, and thighs. You'll need strength in these areas to rock forward and back and to angle your hips for optimal penetration.

**BEST WORKOUT:** Hanging Leg Raises. Using a chinup bar and an overhand grip, hang with your arms straight and shoulder-width apart. Use your abdominal muscles to raise your legs until they're a bit higher than your hips. Hold it for 2 seconds, then return to the starting position. Try for three sets of eight repetitions.

# *Tabletop Sex* *(page 33)*

*Why she likes it: Spontaneous passion, deep penetration.*

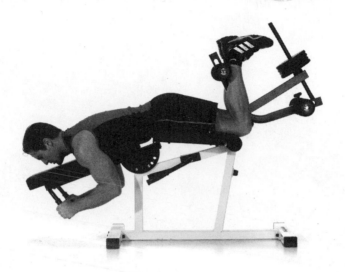

**MUSCLES TO WORK:** Hamstrings. These muscles have to be strong to have sex while standing, especially when you're bent over and thrusting forward.

**BEST WORKOUT:** Leg Curls. Lie facedown on a leg-curl machine. With your hips flat against the bench and your abdominal muscles tight, curl your legs behind you until your feet are about perpendicular to the bench. Pause, then lower your legs slowly to the starting position, stopping just before your knees are straight. Try for three sets of eight repetitions.

# *Sitting* (page 26)

*Why she likes it: Sex while sitting offers the best of all possible worlds. You can penetrate as deeply as you can in lying positions, with a bonus: The woman gets the opportunity to set the pace, moving as quickly or slowly as she likes.*

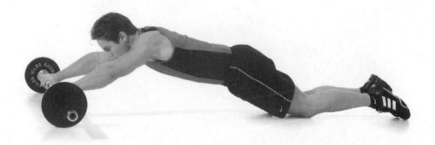

**MUSCLES TO WORK:** Back and abdominals. Strength in these areas makes it easier to hold yourself and your partner upright without fatigue.

**BEST WORKOUT:** Wheel of Torture. Kneel on the floor as though doing a modified pushup, with your hands resting on a barbell. Glide forward as you roll the bar in front of you, flexing your shoulders and extending your spine. Keep going until your hips are in line with your torso. Then slide backward until you're back in the kneeling position. Try for three sets of eight repetitions.

# *Standing, from the Back* (page 30)

*Why she likes it:* Very deep, fast penetration.

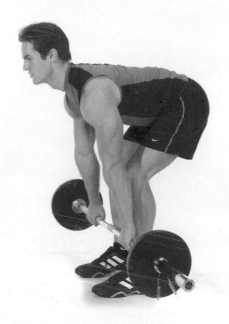

**MUSCLES TO WORK:** Forearms, back, and biceps. You need to hold your partner firmly to keep from thrusting her into a nosedive.

**BEST WORKOUT:** Wide-Stance Romanian Deadlift. Stand with your legs hip-width apart and your knees slightly bent. Grab a barbell with an overhand grip and your hands just beyond shoulder-width apart. Hold the bar at arm's length at mid-thigh level with your shoulders back and chest out. Keeping your back flat and your knees slightly bent, bend forward at the hips, keeping the bar close to your thighs. Lower the bar toward the floor, going as far as you comfortably can. Slowly return to the starting position, keeping your back straight throughout the exercise. Try for three sets of eight repetitions.

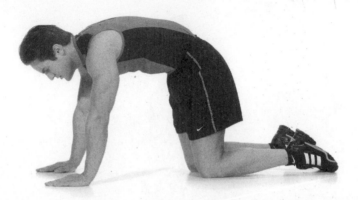

# *Skin the Cat* (page 40)

## *Why she likes it: The giddy headrush.*

**MUSCLES TO WORK:** Deep abdominals. When you're on your knees, and your partner straddles you in an upside-down position, you need strong abdominals to hold yourself upright and to move back and forth.

**BEST WORKOUT:** Kneeling Vacuum. Get down on your hands and knees, keeping your back flat. Take a deep breath, allowing your belly to push out. Then forcibly exhale and round your back as you lift your navel up toward your spine, contracting your pelvic muscles. When you can no longer exhale, keep your back rounded. Hold the contraction for anywhere from 10 to 60 seconds, breathing regularly the whole time. Rest for a minute, then repeat up to 10 times.

# The Honeybee (page 42)

*Why she likes it:* Intense G-spot stimulation with every thrust. This position allows maximum penetration and visual stimulation.

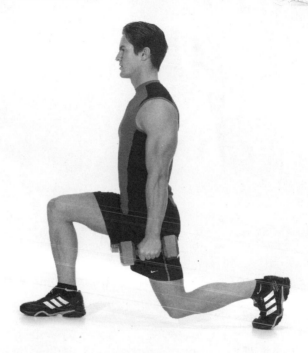

**MUSCLES TO WORK:** Legs, hips, and butt

**BEST WORKOUT:** Dumbbell Lunge. Grab a dumbbell in each hand, your palms facing your body, and stand with your feet hip-width apart. Keeping your back straight, take a long step forward with your right leg. Bend your leg until your right thigh is parallel with the floor. Your left leg should be extended, with your knee slightly bent and almost touching the floor. Keep your right foot stationary as you straighten your right leg. Switch legs and repeat on the other side.

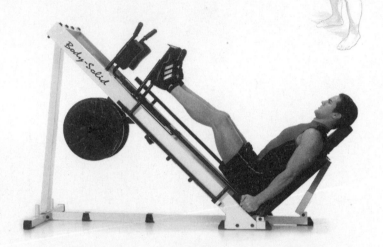

# *Standing* (page 32)

*Why she likes it: Full body-to-body contact, the feel of your hands on her butt.*

**MUSCLES TO WORK:** Calves, hamstrings, and butt. They work together to provide the strength needed to hold your partner off the floor.

**BEST WORKOUT:** Leg Presses, which work all three muscle groups together. Sit on a leg-press machine with your back against the pad and your feet shoulder-width apart on the foot plate. Adjust the seat so your knees are bent slightly more than 90 degrees. Push the weight until your knees are almost locked, then slowly return to the starting position. Try for three sets of eight repetitions.

# *Rear Entry* (page 16)

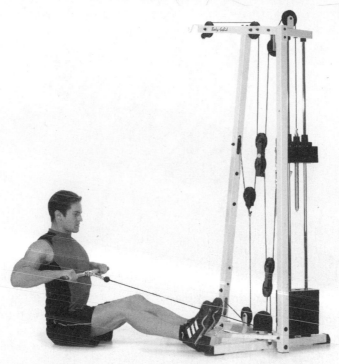

**Why she likes it:** *Rear-entry (or doggy-style) positions allow for very deep penetration and for manual stimulation of her clitoris by either of you.*

**MUSCLES TO WORK:** Back. You need a lot of back strength to hold your partner in position—and to hold yourself upright while thrusting forward.

**BEST WORKOUT:** Cable Seated Row. Sit on the floor, knees bent, and grip the cable handle. Pull the handle straight back until it almost touches your waist; at the same time, pull your shoulders back and push your chest forward. Hold for a moment, then extend your arms as you return to the starting position; your shoulders and lower back should flex forward slightly. Try for three sets of eight repetitions.

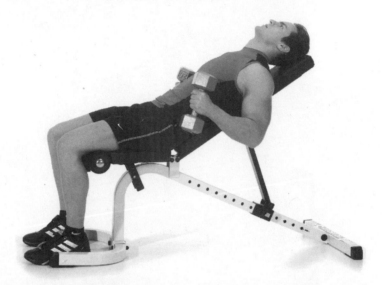

# *Side by Side* *(page 22)*

**Why she likes it:** *There's deep penetration in the spooning variation of the side-by-side position, it's easy for you (or her) to touch her clitoris, and it involves little vigorous thrusting—good when you're both tired.*

**MUSCLES TO WORK:** Arms. The penis tends to slip from the vagina with some frequency in this position. You need strong arms to grasp her pelvis and hold her tight.

**BEST WORKOUT:** Incline Hammer Curl. Sit back on an incline bench with about a 45-degree angle. Hold a dumbbell in each hand, with your arms hanging at your sides. With your palms facing inward and your upper arms still, curl the dumbbells straight up, keeping your wrists locked. You can work both arms simultaneously or, if that's too difficult, alternate arms. Try for two or three sets of eight repetitions each.

## *Scissors* (*page 46*)

***Why she likes it:*** *Her clitoris will get extra stimulation as it rubs against your inner thigh during thrusting in this crisscross position.*

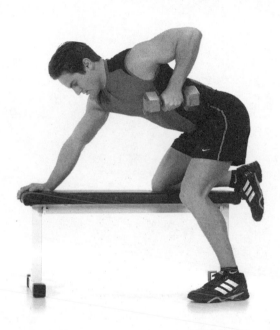

**MUSCLES TO WORK:** Latissimus dorsi (back muscles). A strong back makes it easier to hold her close when you're in a sitting position.

**BEST WORKOUT:** One-Arm Dumbbell Row. Holding a dumbbell in your left hand, rest your right knee and right hand on a bench. Keep your back flat as you let the dumbbell hang down to your side so your arm lines up just in front of your shoulder. With your left foot firmly on the floor, knee slightly bent, pull the dumbbell up and in toward your torso, raising it as high as it will go. Try for three sets of eight repetitions, then switch positions and work the other arm.

## *The Pretzel* (*page 54*)

*Why she likes it:* Access to her clitoris in a comfortable reclining position.

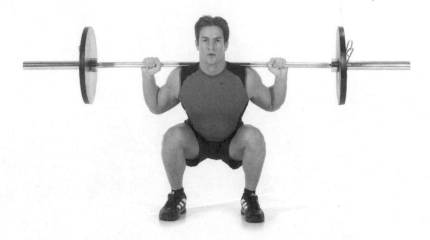

**MUSCLES TO WORK:** Butt. You have to have strong glutes to hold this position.

**BEST WORKOUT:** Barbell squats. Place a barbell at shoulder level on a squat rack. Grip the bar with your hands slightly more than shoulder-width apart, palms facing front. Step under the bar so that it's evenly positioned across your upper back and shoulders, not your neck. Stand up straight, with your feet hip-width apart and your knees slightly bent. Don't drop your head; keep it in line with your torso. Keeping your feet flat and torso straight, bend your knees slightly and squat down, as though sitting in a chair behind you. Don't allow your knees to extend past your toes. Continue moving downward until your thighs are parallel to the floor. Then slowly rise to a standing position. Try for three sets of eight repetitions.

# CHAPTER 7

# YOUR BEATING HEART: THE CARDIOVASCULAR KEY TO GOOD SEX

**ATHLETES IN FULL-CONTACT SPORTS CAN COUNT ON TRAINERS TO PUMP THEM FULL OF OXYGEN OR MASSAGE THEIR MUSCLES WHEN THEY'RE ON THE BRINK OF COLLAPSE.** Sad to say, you can't get the same kind of help if your body suddenly gives out in the bedroom. If you like the idea of having sex all night, get used to the idea that your successes or failures are entirely up to you.

*"There is nothing more embarrassing than panting and gasping when performing even the simplest moves,"* a 24-year-old computer support specialist in Montclair, New Jersey, told us. *"I almost always get tired and have to rest,"* added a 52-year-old technical writer.

Here's a simple fact about the human male: He needs air. If you can't breathe, you can't make love, at least not very well. Guys who are out of shape may notice that they can't have sex and talk at the same time. They have trouble when they try to talk *and* have sex *and* change positions a few times.

There are all sorts of solutions to the kinds of sexual problems that pain men most, such as coming too quickly or not getting hard (or hard enough) when they want to. These are critical issues that deserve all the attention they get. But the foundation, the *heart* of good sex always comes down to air. Vigorous sex requires endurance no less than an erection. If your cardiovascular system can't cut it, neither will you.

More is involved than just kissing and breathing at the same time. Your entire body pays the price if your heart and lungs don't work at peak capacity.

▶ A lot of muscles come into play when you have sex. Each of them requires an abundant flow of oxygen. Limit the amount of air that comes in—and the amount of carbon dioxide that's carted out—and your strength will plummet. You'll tire easily. You'll be more likely to get debilitating, sex-stopping cramps.

▶ Blood flows to the most active muscles when you're having sex. At the same time, it continues to circulate to other body systems. If your heart isn't pounding efficiently, circulation can be significantly compromised. No, you won't die (probably), but there may be a drop in the system-wide distribution of nutrients, hormones, or other key chemicals that you need for full energy and arousal.

▶ The landmark Massachusetts Male Aging Study, which tracked more than 600 middle-age and older men for more than 10 years, found that those who weren't active had twice the risk of impotence compared with those who took a brisk, 2-mile walk daily. Another study, this one at the New England Research Institute in Watertown, Massachusetts, reported that 31 percent of sedentary men developed impotence, compared with only 9 percent who whipped their cardiovascular systems into shape.

No matter how much you lift weights, no matter how many games of golf you play, no matter how often you sort through all the clothes that you've heaped on the now-invisible exercise bike, you have to add cardiovascular workouts into your life. You'll notice that we didn't say that you might want to think about it. You *have* to do it—to save your sex life as well as your life.

Stamina originates with a strong heart. The best way to strengthen the heart is with aerobic workouts: jogging, fast walking,

## CAN A MAN FAKE AN ORGASM?

Of course. Men can fake anything. Unlike a woman's orgasm, however, men leave a little something behind. Even if your partner doesn't feel the spurt of semen—and many women don't—she's bound to notice something's amiss.

A better question to ask yourself is why you'd even want to fake an orgasm. It's true that women (and men) sometimes fake orgasms to make their partners feel better or simply to end a sexual session for whatever reason. But this kind of deception, however well intentioned, isn't as harmless as it appears. Once you start faking anything, and once you get caught (as you will eventually), your partner will start wondering what else you lie about. Maybe, her thinking might go, you're not really attracted to her. Maybe you just pretend to like her in bed. Maybe you just pretend to like her, *period*.

Faking an orgasm might be a time-honored way to let your partner (and yourself) off the hook, but the possible repercussions aren't worth it. Besides, you want to have the kind of relationship that fosters sexual openness, not deceit. Who cares if you (or your partner) don't come on occasion? It's normal. Why lie about it?

swimming, cycling, and so on. Any time you kick your heart rate up a few notches and keep it there for half an hour or so, your heart muscle gets stronger, and your resting heart rate declines. The lungs get more efficient. Blood pressure goes down. Circulation goes up. And on and on.

*"I started running a few years ago, and my endurance went way up. Believe it or not, I have better erections now than I did when I was 30 because I don't party any more, and I work out regularly,"* a 45-year-old contractor in Tucson told us.

*"I meet a lot more women than I used to, probably because my body image and confidence is a lot higher since I started aerobic training,"* says a 23-year-old student in Madison, Wisconsin.

What else can you get from regular cardiovascular training? Take a look.

▶ **An increase in sex drive.** A study of more than 8,000 people ages 18 to 45 found that 40 percent had increases in sexual arousal after starting a regular exercise program. One-third of them reported that they had sex more often.

▶ **Better orgasms.** Researchers at the University of California report that sedentary middle-age men who started exercising for 1 hour three times weekly had better orgasms, better erections, and higher overall sexual satisfaction.

▶ **More testosterone.** Aerobic workouts stimulate the body's production of testosterone, the hormone that stimulates libido and promotes erections.

▶ **Less fat.** Sure, you can lose weight (or at least fat) by lifting weights, but it's a slow way to do it. Cardiovascular training puts you on the fast track. Men who walk at a leisurely, 4-mile-an-hour pace for 30 minutes will burn about 240 calories, 40 percent of which come from fat. Men who exercise more vigorously can count on burning lard at up to *eight times* the normal rate.

▶ **Less death.** Well, that's a bit of a stretch, but cardiovascular conditioning dramatically reduces the risk of heart attack, the leading cause of death in American men and women. It also cuts the risk of diabetes and colon cancer as well as high blood pressure.

▶ **A better mood.** The brain churns out endorphins, opiate-like brain chemicals that make you feel calm and self-assured, when you kick-start your cardiovascular system. The same chemicals that account for the runner's high can cut your risk of depression and anxiety while boosting levels of confidence and self-esteem.

## WHY AEROBICS?

The terms *aerobics* and *aerobic exercise* are often used interchangeably, but they aren't quite the same thing. Aerobics generally refers to aerobic dance—leotards, mirrored walls, and nerve-grating, upbeat music. Aerobic exercise, by contrast, means any exercise that gets your heart pumping faster than usual—and keeps it at that rate for an extended period.

Strictly speaking, any activity performed faster than sitting in a chair is aerobic. But to produce any real benefit, there has to be substantial physical effort involved—which is why you won't see billiard players on the Olympic medal stand any time in the near future. True aerobic exercise, the kinds of workouts that tax your heart and lungs as well as your muscles, requires that you push yourself to roughly 60 to 90 percent of your maximum ability. More simply, you get an aerobic workout—also known as cardiovascular exercise—when you significantly raise your heartbeat for at least 30 minutes at a stretch.

Not so long ago, nearly everyone earned their daily crust through hard, physical labor. Aerobic workouts were pretty much a given. Lately, though, we've all gotten more sedentary. If you spend your days doing nothing more physically taxing than fingering computer keys, and your nightly activity is jamming buttons on the remote control, you can bet that your heart and lungs aren't doing what they should—and your sex life, including your ability to even *want* a sex life, is probably paying the price.

Scientists first started examining the link between physical activity and the heart in the 1960s. Harvard and Stanford scientists discovered that longshoremen who were promoted to management positions developed heart disease at a much higher rate than the guys who stayed on the dock. They surmised that hard physical activity had significant cardio-protecting effects—and decades of subsequent research proved them right.

▼

**Men in some African tribes run while maintaining erections. They believe that it increases sexual stamina.**

▲

For a long time, researchers were pretty sure that cardiovascular workouts had a significant health edge over non-aerobic types of exercise, such as weight lifting or short sprints. There's no question that you really have to push the heart and lungs to achieve true cardiovascular fitness. For cardiovascular *health*, however, you don't have to sweat anywhere near as hard as people once thought. Almost any kind of exercise, even leisurely walking, can extend your life and reduce the risk of diabetes, high blood pressure, and other diseases. But the basic premise of cardiovascular training is still true: Pushing your heart and lungs past their usual comfort zones can extend your life *and* improve your sex life.

When you engage in any kind of exercise—anything from mowing the grass to making love—muscle cells are suddenly stressed. Roused from their lassitude, they demand a quick infusion of blood and oxygen. The heart responds by pumping harder and faster in order to route more blood through the lungs for oxygenation. As long as the exercise continues, the muscles continuously demand more blood, and the heart and lungs keep working at an accelerated rate.

The heart, keep in mind, is a muscle, one that gets stronger the harder you work it. As the heart gets more buffed, it starts doing the same amount of work with less effort. That's why men who work out tend to have lower resting heart rates than those who are sedentary.

The blood vessels get stronger and more elastic when you start cardiovascular training. Circulation improves throughout the body, including in the tiny blood vessels that carry blood through the penis and make erections possible. Men who start almost any kind of cardiovascular training have better bloodflow with lower blood pressure. They're less likely to develop the kinds of vascular disease that can put their sex lives out of commission. And they're more likely to have the extra energy and libido that can push their erotic pleasures to another level.

## THE AEROBIC BOTTOM LINE

The President's Council on Fitness has identified four essential components—the ABCDs—of cardiovascular fitness.

▶ Amount. For optimal fitness, strive for a workout intensity that pushes your heart rate to 65 to 85 percent of its maximum capacity. We'll talk more about this in just a bit. In the meantime, don't let the numbers throw you. You can ballpark it by exercising with an intensity somewhere between fairly light and fairly hard. Even if you don't quite hit the target range, you'll get nearly all of the benefits, minus a percentage point or two.

▶ Best type. This one's easy. The best aerobic workout is one that you'll actually do. Doesn't matter if it's jumping rope, swimming laps, or running hard a few steps ahead of the IRS. If you do it regularly, you'll get fit.

▶ Consistency. Good intentions don't count. For optimal sexual (and physical and emotional) health, you need to set aside time 3 to 5 days a week. Don't expect to get the same benefits if you blow off your workouts for 3 weeks, then pound yourself into a frenzy a few days in a row. Consistency is everything—and that goes for downtime as well. When you're starting out, plan on resting for a day or two between workouts. Time off is especially important if you're running or doing other high-impact activities.

▶ Duration. Plan on exercising for 30 to 60 minutes each time. That's a huge range, of course, but it doesn't seem to matter all that much exactly where in the range you fall. Recent studies show that men can get nearly the same health benefits from a 30-minute workout as they can from a full hour.

Since the core of any aerobic workout requires boosting the heart rate above its usual level, it's worth taking a little time to explain exactly what this means—and how to customize your workouts to shove your heart into the optimal zone.

Optimal, incidentally, doesn't mean "the most you can do before you die." Don't launch into cardiovascular training with the idea that your heart needs to be beating so hard that it bulges from your chest; that sweat should be spouting from every pore; and that your head will be pounding as though it's about to explode, either shortly before or after you pass out.

With the possible exception of Richard Simmons videos, aerobic workouts shouldn't be painful. You simply need to elevate your heartbeat until it reaches what is known as your target heart rate. This isn't defined by the outer limits of your heart's endurance. Rather, it represents your aerobic range—roughly 60 to 90 percent of the maximum rate your heart is capable of. (Although the President's Council recommends 65 to 85 percent, 60 to 90 percent is more realistic.)

A huge amount of research has shown that this is the ideal exercise range. For example, researchers at the University of California in San Diego looked at 78 healthy but sedentary men. Some were assigned to a "couch group" to act as controls. The others enrolled in a 9-month program of aerobic exercise in which the intensity of the workouts—walking at a moderate pace for 60 minutes 4 days a week—pushed their hearts into the aerobic range.

Men in the exercise group not only reported having more sex than those who were sedentary, they also enjoyed it more. And the more they exercised, the better the sex got.

Every man has a different target heart rate. The easiest way to identify your personal range is to subtract your age from 220 and multiply that by 0.6 to get the lower end of the range, then again by 0.9 to get the upper figure.

If you're 40, for example, you'd first subtract your age from 220 (answer: 180). Multiply that by 0.6 to get 108. That's the lower end of your aerobic range. Now, start again. Multiply 180 by 0.9 to get 162. That's the upper end of your range. Now you know what you're shooting for.

Just to make things a little more complicated, studies have shown that people who've been sedentary for a lot of years can improve their aerobic fitness by starting with a target heart rate as low as 40 percent of max. This time, subtract your age from 220 and multiply that number by 0.4. Once you're in better shape, you can kick it up into the 60 to 90 percent range.

Checking your pulse isn't the only way to rate the intensity of aerobic exercise. Here are some other options.

▶ A heart-rate monitor. They're easy to use, inexpensive if you don't get all the bells and whistles, and available at just about any sporting goods store.

▶ The talk test. This is one of the best techniques because there are no equations, no stopping to check your pulse, and almost no thought. All you have to do is ask yourself if you have enough wind during exercise to talk at the same time. As you might expect, scientists have given this technique its own gaudy name: the Talk Test Method (TTM). It can be quite

## FEELING THE BEAT

Forget what you see on *ER:* Taking an accurate pulse isn't always easy, especially during exercise, when your chest is heaving, and you're sucking every bit of air you can muster. Here's the easiest way to do it.

▶ Locate the carotid artery, the big pipe in your neck that runs alongside the windpipe and Adam's apple. If you look closely, you'll see it pulsing with each beat.

▶ Put your finger on the artery so you can feel the pulse. Count the beats for 10 seconds, then multiply that number by six. That's your heart rate per minute. Pressing too hard on the artery will skew the count. Also, don't use your thumb; it has its own pulse, which can complicate things.

▶ Take the reading within 10 seconds of pausing during exercise. If you wait longer than that, your heart rate will drop quickly. You may think you're not exercising hard enough, when in fact you may have reached your target heart range or even gone beyond it. Pushing yourself beyond that range is neither necessary nor safe.

useful in determining your aerobic comfort zone, particularly when you're just starting out. If you're able to talk during your workout without a great deal of strain, you're most likely in your comfort zone.

▶ Borg Rating of Perceived Exertion. It's a useful measure of exercise intensity because it basically rates how you feel. On a scale of 10, the average man engaged in aerobic exercise should rate his physical and mental fatigue somewhere between 4 and 6. The scale looks something like this:

0–1: No exertion. You're either watching TV, sleeping, or dead. Breathing is so slight, it's barely noticeable.

2–3: Minimal exertion. For example, working on the computer (non-porn sites only) or easy walking. Breathing is normal, and conversation is easy.

4–5: Moderate exertion. Jogging or fast walking, for example. Breathing is getting harder.

6–7: Very strong exertion. You might be running, cycling, or swimming. Breathing is heavy.

8–9: Close to maximum exertion. Sprinting will get you there. You're struggling to breathe.

10: Maximum exertion. This would be an all-out sprint. You're absolutely at your limit.

It's worth mentioning that all of these techniques and numbers apply only to men in good health. If you're 40 years or older or have risk factors for heart disease (such as smoking or high cholesterol), talk to your doctor before starting any kind of exercise plan. You might be advised to take it far slower than the guidelines advise, at least until you get into better shape.

## DESIGN YOUR WORKOUT

As we mentioned earlier, you have to pick a cardiovascular workout that you really and truly enjoy. Otherwise, you'll find it hard to get out of bed in the morning, much less out the door. Of course, it's possible that you don't even *need* to add exercise to your life. If you live in a cozy home in rural Vermont, for example, and you spend your days cutting, hauling, and stacking firewood to fend off the brutal cold, you're probably already getting all the aerobic exercise that you need. The same if you live in a 20th-floor walk-up in New York City, and you go up and down the stairs a dozen times a day.

Most of us, though, need some kind of "artificial" exercise. What's it to be? Walking? Jogging? Running? Swimming? Prize-fighting? Sure, they're all good. So are a million other things. Walking fast to the supermarket instead of driving. Loping along behind the lawnmower. It doesn't matter what you do, as long as it kicks your heart into the target range and keeps it there for at least 30 minutes. Your heart doesn't know the difference between "real" exercise and simply moving quickly.

If you've practiced exercise avoidance most of your life, you'll obviously want to start slowly. More than a few guys haul themselves off the couch, go out and spend $1,000 on a new bike, then irritate the heck out of their friends when they call from the next county needing a ride home. Moving too quickly into exercise will only cause fatigue, sore muscles, and mental and physical burnout.

So where do you start? Just in case you're wondering, sex probably won't do it. Yes, it provides a vigorous workout. But unless you can keep it up for 30 minutes three or four times a week, stopping periodically to take your pulse to ensure you're in the target range, you'd better not count on it. Here are some more practical options.

**DO IT WITH CLASS.** Just about every health club offers a range of cardiovascular workout classes. Traditional aerobics classes were dominated by women, and many still are—but don't assume that they're lightweight. Just about any class will give you a killer workout. If the so-called aerobic dance workouts aren't for you, you have other options: Spinning, aero-boxing (or plain boxing), and jump-roping, to name a few. They're often geared to men, although plenty of women take them, too.

**GO UP A LEVEL.** How many times have you walked right past the stairs at your apartment complex or office? You're ignoring one of the best aerobic workouts you can get. Climbing stairs—and coming back down—puts tremendous strain on the quadriceps, hamstring, butt, hip, and calf muscles. It puts an equally hard strain on the heart and lungs. In fact, researchers say that the exertion of sex is the equivalent of climbing stairs, so you can think of it as a kind of training.

Best of all, stairclimbing is free. No membership fees, no fancy clothes, and no waiting in line when linebacker-size dudes form packs around the dumbbell rack.

**RIDE YOURSELF RAGGED.** Cycling is a great workout for the legs, lungs, and heart. More and more men are doing it, either on the road or in Spinning classes, because it's a lot easier on the knees and back than running. It's also more fun than a lot of other aerobic workouts, which is probably why men who take up a cycling program tend to stick with it.

**GET YOUR OARS WET.** If you're lucky enough to live in an area with a lake or river, rowing, also known as sculling, is probably the best cardiovascular workout you can get. A NASA study found that rowing consistently burns 15 to 20 percent more calories than cycling—and you don't have to worry about flat tires.

The rowing machines at gyms are good substitutes, especially those with sliding seats. They'll quickly build your back, arms, butt, and legs and provide a tough workout for your heart and lungs as well.

**GIVE RUNNING ANOTHER CHANCE.** It's true that millions of men have tried running, and an almost equal number hate it. The reason for running's spotty reputation is that too many men go all out. They force themselves to run longer, faster, and harder and eventually collapse with blasted knees—or at least get sick of the chronically sore ankles, shins, and feet that seem almost inevitable.

But if you run smart—that is, staying below the threshold of fatigue and soreness—running is a superb workout. Even running at a sedate, 12-minute-mile pace will burn roughly 10 calories a minute. Then there's the simplicity factor. You don't have to learn a lot about technique. Just put one foot in front of the other.

Running does put a lot of stress on your body. Each time your foot hits the ground, it strikes with a force equal to three to four times your body weight. You have to be sensible—by running on grass, for example; replacing your shoes every 3 to 6 months; and warming up before runs and cooling down after.

**GET IN THE SWIM.** Swimming is easier on the back, ligaments, and joints than running. It burns a tremendous amount of calories. It requires you to use just about all of your major muscle groups, while stimulating the cardiovascular system at an impressive level. Water gives 12 times the resistance of air, which is why a 180-pound guy can burn 630 calories an hour doing a slow crawl—about the same as running for an hour on hilly terrain.

The water isn't our natural environment, of course, and swimming takes some practice to achieve a reasonable level of expertise. Definitely consider getting qualified instruction if you aren't a natural. Invest in good goggles to minimize the chlorine sting. And give some thought to the suit you'll be comfortable in. A standard-issue racing suit offers virtually no drag in the water, but it will reveal parts of your anatomy that only your intimates are familiar with. The standard beach britches work fine for most guys.

**TAKE A WALK.** It's never been accorded much respect by the more macho exercise elements, but look at the facts. Men who walk at a moderate pace get the same cardiovascular benefits as those who jog. Then there's the injury factor: It doesn't happen when you walk. If you can get up from the couch, you can walk. No trainers or specialized gear needed.

Walking does take time, though, a scarce commodity in today's world. To get the best results, you'll probably want to walk for about 45 minutes most days of the week. Why not make it fun? Take your dog. Use the time to catch up with your friends. Meet women at the park. You're going to be out there anyway; you might as well enjoy it.

**TRY WALKING-PLUS.** True, walking is a superb way to ease into an aerobic workout program. It's easy to do; it's easy on the joints; it's easy to enjoy. On the other hand, it doesn't exactly get your adrenaline pumping. Some men enjoy the mental peace they get from walking. Others, within a few weeks, find that they're bored out of their minds.

Part of the problem is that men tend to approach walking as a pleasant stroll. That's good for enjoyment, and it's okay for your heart. Okay, but not great. The only way to transform a stroll into a heart-pounding, 30- to 45-minute workout is to pump it up.

▶ Walk slowly for 5 to 10 minutes to warm up.

▶ Pick up your pace to 4 to 5 miles an hour. You should be swinging your arms, not letting them dangle at your sides. After a few minutes, you should be breathing harder, and your heart rate will be picking up.

▼

**A modest pucker utilizes two facial muscles, but a full-fledged, passionate kiss employs 34. Result: A 1-minute kiss burns roughly 26 calories.**

▲

▶ Choose a route that includes some hills. Walking at an angle stresses the muscles in different ways and increases the rush of blood through the heart and lungs.

▶ Pick up the pace some more. Again, you want to be breathing hard, but not so hard that you're sucking air. Remember the rule we mentioned earlier: Your breathing should be labored, yet you should have sufficient reserves to talk at the same time.

▶ Kick into a gentle jog, somewhere between fast walking and running. After a few minutes of that, increase your pace to a full jog. That's where you're going to stay for the duration of your outing. You don't want to break into a run, because it's hard on the joints. A steady jog will take you along at a speed that's two to three times faster than when you started.

▶ Slow down for the last few minutes of your route. Slow from a jog to fast walking, and then to a leisurely stroll. This cooldown time gives your heart and lungs a chance to recover, and it flushes lactic acid from your leg muscles.

Men who stick to a walking-plus program usually find that their resting heart rates have significantly slowed within a few weeks. The needle on the scale won't swing quite as far to the right. You'll have toned your body as well as your lungs. And you'll probably find that you have more strength and endurance in the bedroom because your overall energy has spiked upward. Ultimately, that's what this is all about.

## INTERVAL TRAINING

Aerobic training is terrific for cardiovascular health, but it's not so great at building strength or burning fat. Sure, you can have great sex if you're overweight, and you hardly need the muscles of a pro wrestler to play with most positions. But a man who's lean is generally more attractive to women—and a man who *feels* lean and confident will definitely get more attention. The trick is to add fuel to your usual aerobic workouts with a technique known as interval training—slipping high-intensity exercises into your normal routine.

The idea is simple enough. Whatever level of exercise you're accustomed to eventually becomes routine; progress slows or stops. Trainers call this phase a plateau, and it's frustrating because all of your hard work doesn't seem to be adding up to much. The only way to break through the plateau is to give your body challenges it hasn't had before.

With interval training, you alternate bouts of vigorous, *anaerobic* exercise with your usual aerobic sessions. Here's an example. Suppose you've been running for a few months—nothing crazy, but solid and consistent. It's become as easy as breathing. Your muscles aren't challenged, your lungs aren't challenged, and your mind definitely isn't challenged. So you throw a little extra something into the mix—say, periodic sprints that stress the muscles in a way that routine running doesn't. The added stress tears down muscle fibers. They're forced to rebuild themselves, which translates into an increase in strength and size.

Another benefit of interval training is that it promotes faster weight loss. Aerobic workouts do burn fat, but only after you've already burned your available supply of carbohydrates—and the benefits stop when the exercise does. When you throw an anaerobic workout into the mix, you burn fat right away and keep burning it even after exercise is over. At the same time, the stressed muscles continue the rebuilding process even when you're lounging on the couch.

Here are the basics.

▶ Several times a week, intersperse your regular workout—jogging, cycling, whatever—with high-intensity, strength-building exertion.

▶ The aerobic part of your workout should be done at an intensity of 50 to 70 percent of your target heart rate. The anaerobic phase should kick you into the 80 to 90 percent range. (Check with your doctor before pushing your exercise intensity to these maximum levels.)

▶ The anaerobic phase of your workouts should last 2 to 10 minutes. Continue interspersing bursts of high-intensity exercise. For example, walk or jog at your usual steady pace for 2 minutes. Then walk or run hard for 2 minutes. Then switch back to the slower pace. Repeat each interval eight times.

▶ Allow yourself plenty of rest during interval training. If you're getting winded or sore, take a break for a few minutes, then resume your exercise.

▶ Always start with a warmup. For example, start out by walking for 5 to 10 minutes, keeping your heart rate at about 50 to 60 percent of its target range. Then increase the intensity to your usual level and from there, kick in with the intervals.

## THE COOLDOWN PHASE

Trainers always advise men to end aerobic workouts with a cooldown period, and men just as often ignore them. Yes, it takes a couple of minutes that you'd probably rather use for something else, and yes, it's a little on the boring side. Do it anyway. Stopping suddenly after hard exercise puts unnecessary strain on the heart. You can pass out if your blood pressure

## UNSEXY SMOKING

It wasn't that long ago that the US government supplied soldiers with free packs of Lucky Strikes, and lab-coated physicians appeared on television commercials to extol the health benefits of charcoal-filtered Larks. For a long time, cigarettes were considered the pinnacle of class and sophistication.

We know today, of course, that smoking is a dangerous habit, one that kills an estimated 400,000 Americans a year. We won't hammer you with the litany of risks; you know them all by heart. Suffice it to say that smoking is a common cause of impotence. Chemicals in the smoke cause blood vessels to clamp down. Less blood means you won't get as hard as you should, if you even get hard at all. Smoking even makes the erectile tissue in the penis less sensitive to stimulation.

If you're a smoker and are thinking about trying to quit, well, you have our sympathy. The tobacco habit is even harder to kick than heroin. There are plenty of stop-smoking approaches that can make it a little easier. Patches, for example, suffuse your body with nicotine while you try to beat the habit. Nicotine gum is another option. There are also drugs such as Zyban (bupropion) that can minimize cravings.

Once you quit, you have about a 3-day window of real suffering. That's about how long it takes to clear your body of the physical addiction to nicotine. After that, the craving is mainly psychological. Your body is no longer hooked, but all of your habits—having a smoke with your morning coffee, for example—will do everything in their power to drag you back in. This psychological craving is the toughest to beat.

People who say it's easy to quit have obviously never smoked. It is hard—quite possibly the hardest thing you've ever done. Do it anyway. If you fail the first time, as you probably will, keep trying. Don't hesitate to ask your doctor for help. When you quit, you'll have the satisfaction of knowing you'll live longer. You'll have more energy, you'll breathe better, and you'll have a better time in bed. Go for it.

drops too far. And you'll almost certainly have pain later because you didn't take the time to flush out the lactic acid that accumulates during exercise.

At the end of your workout, take about 5 minutes to cool down with slow, easy exercise. Walk slowly after a hard jog—or jog slowly after a hard run. Cycle at a breathe-easy pace. Do some stretches and breathe deeply. All you're trying to do at this point is avoid shocking your system and keep blood from pooling in your legs and feet.

## PROGRAMS YOU CAN USE

There are as many effective cardiovascular training programs as there are men to invent them. Since just about any activity, done quickly, puts beneficial stress on the heart and lungs, and since every man enjoys different things, the potential permutations are endless. But we've gone ahead and created a few basic, ready-to-go programs to make it easier: one for beginners, one for intermediate exercisers, and one for the hard-core contingent.

### CARDIOVASCULAR TRAINING, PHASE 1

If you're just starting to get in shape, plan on three cardiovascular sessions a week, using a technique known as continuous training. In other words, pick one cardiovascular exercise and do it for the full duration of your workout. You can do anything you want on different days, but make each day consistent. For example, ride a stationary bike, swim, or fast-walk for 30 to 45 minutes at a pop, making sure that your target heart rate clocks in at around 50 to 60 percent of your top capacity for at least 20 minutes of the workout.

Incidentally, don't be surprised if you notice a sudden drop in energy once you launch into your program. This is normal. Within a few weeks, you'll rebound to your previous level, then surpass it.

▶ **MONDAY:** 10-minute warmup; 20 minutes of continuous exercise; 5-minute cooldown.

▶ **TUESDAY:** Take the day off. And quit complaining: It wasn't that bad.

▶ **WEDNESDAY:** 10-minute warmup; 20 minutes of continuous exercise; 5-minute cooldown.

▶ **THURSDAY:** Rest.

▶ **FRIDAY:** 10 minute warmup; 20 minutes of continuous exercise; 5-minute cooldown.

▶ **SATURDAY** and **SUNDAY**: Rest.

## CARDIOVASCULAR TRAINING, PHASE 2

▼

**Most men who start a cardiovascular training program can expect to lose at least 1 pound a week.**

▲

This workout is designed for men who are in pretty good shape. If you've stuck with Phase 1 of the program for a few months or are otherwise active, it's time to push yourself. Here, the workout intensity is higher. You'll want to increase your target heart rate to 60 to 75 percent of your top capacity. You'll also work out more—4 or 5 days a week instead of 3.

You'll also notice that the workout is more varied. On each day of exercise, do something different: running, swimming, biking, climbing stairs, whatever. We've given exercise examples—but they're just that. Feel free to replace them with whatever aerobic activity you like best.

▶ **MONDAY:** 10-minute warmup; 25 minutes of continuous exercise—say, biking—at 70 percent of your maximum heart rate; 10-minute cooldown.

▶ **TUESDAY:** Rest.

▶ **WEDNESDAY:** 10-minute warmup; swim for 35 minutes at 70 percent of your maximum heart rate; 10-minute cooldown.

▶ **THURSDAY:** 10 minute warmup; bike for 45 minutes at 60 percent of your maximum heart rate; 5-minute cooldown.

▶ **FRIDAY:** Rest.

▶ **SATURDAY:** Do a shorter, higher-intensity workout: 10 minute warmup at 50 percent of your maximum heart rate; 20 minutes on the bike at 75 percent; 10-minute cooldown.

▶ **SUNDAY:** Rest. Or repeat Saturday's workout.

## CARDIOVASCULAR TRAINING, PHASE 3

Make no mistake: This is a tough workout. Don't try it unless you've been getting regular aerobic exercise for about a year. As with Phase 2, do whatever exercises you like best.

▶ **MONDAY:** 10-minute warmup; 45 minutes of exercise at 75 percent of your maximum heart rate; 10-minute cooldown.

▶ **TUESDAY:** 15-minute warmup at 50 to 60 percent of your maximum heart rate; 50 minutes of exercise at 70 to 75 percent; 5-minute cooldown.

▶ **WEDNESDAY:** 10-minute warmup at 50 to 60 percent; spend the next 20 minutes switching between hard (90 percent of your maximum heart rate) and moderate (50 percent) exercise, alternating every 2 minutes; 10-minute cooldown.

▶ **THURSDAY:** Rest.

▶ **FRIDAY:** 10-minute warmup at 50 to 60 percent of your maximum heart rate; 20 minutes of exercise at 80 percent; 10-minute cooldown.

▶ **SATURDAY:** 10-minute warmup at 50 to 60 percent; 50 minutes of exercise at 70 to 75 percent; throw in 10 minutes of hard biking, swimming, running, or whatever in your routine; 5-minute cooldown.

▶ **SUNDAY:** Rest.

# INDEX

Masturbation *(cont.)*
  for sensual pleasure, 74,
    92–93
  in Tantric sex, 92–93
Medical treatment for sexual
    problems, 71
Medications and erection
    impairment, 72
Mini-orgasms, 85, 100
Missionary position. *See*
    Man-on-top sex position
Mood, cardiovascular training
    for improving, 231
Multiple orgasms, <u>60</u>, 84–85,
    100
Muscle makeup and strength
    training, 151

**N**

Neck stretching exercise, 132,
    **132**
Nicotine gum, <u>245</u>
Nicotine patches, <u>245</u>

**O**

On-bended-knee sex position,
    50, **50–51**
Orgasms. *See also* Ejaculation
  bigasm, <u>60</u>
  cardiovascular training and,
    230
  contractile phase, 85
  delaying
    anxiety about, 90
    habit and, 91
    improving ability, tips for,
      73–75
    Kegels and, 76–79
    pull-out-and-stop
      technique, 100

    sexual response cycle and,
      going through, 73
    stop-and-go technique, 99
    stop-and-squeeze
      technique, 74–75, 77,
      85, 99
    taoist advice, 100–101
    tense-and-tease technique,
      99–100
  faking, <u>229</u>
  Kegel exercises and, 76–79
  mini, 85, 100
  multiple, <u>60</u>, 84–85, 100
  penis before, 96
  perspective on, whimsical,
    34
  refraining from, in Tantric
    sex, <u>90</u>
  sensation of, 73, 89
  in sexual response of men,
    89, **89**
  time needed to reach, 67
  trigasm, <u>60</u>
  visualization and, 97–98
  "white light," 94
  women's, <u>87</u>
Oxytocin, 36

**P**

Patches, nicotine, <u>245</u>
PC muscle, 77, 84–85, 100
Pelvic exercises
  benefits of, 79
  Horse Stance, 83, **83**
  Pelvic Bounce, 81, **81**
  Pelvic Lift, 80, **80**
  Pelvic Tilt, 82, **82**
Pelvis and sex, 79
Penis
  anatomy of, 69–71, **69**
  bloodflow and, 69–71